ROCKFORD PUBLIC LIBRARY
3 1112 01519775 5

Y0-BGW-664

J 612.86 EXT
Extreme stinkers

080307

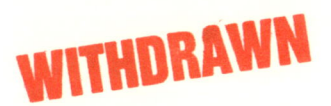

WITHDRAWN

ROCKFORD PUBLIC LIBRARY
Rockford, Illinois
www.rockfordpubliclibrary.org
815-965-9511

EXTREME STINKERS

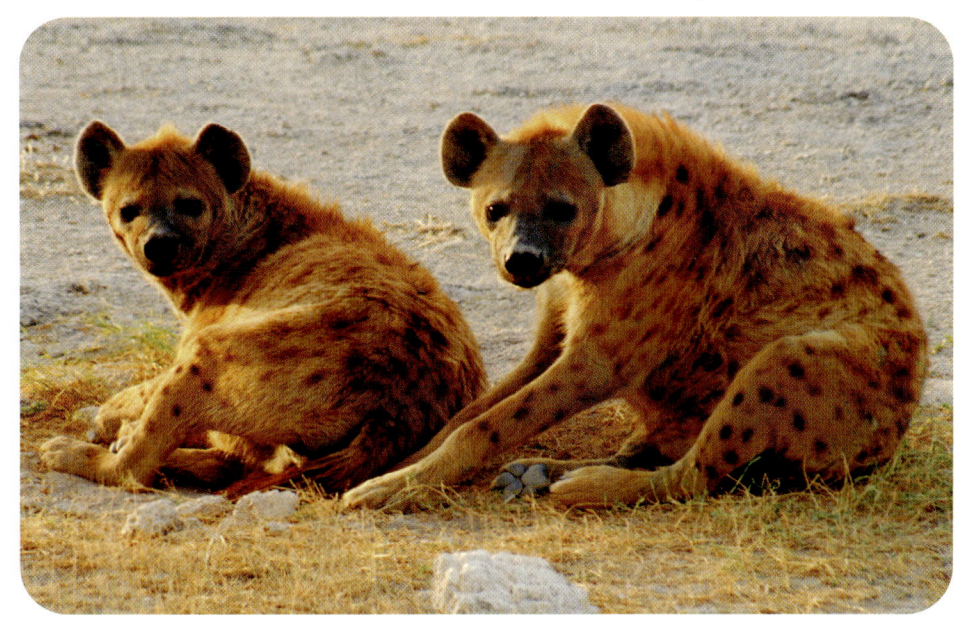

BLACKBIRCH PRESS
An imprint of Thomson Gale, a part of The Thomson Corporation

THOMSON
GALE

Detroit • New York • San Francisco • San Diego • New Haven, Conn. • Waterville, Maine • London • Munich

THOMSON
GALE

© 2005 Thomson Gale, a part of The Thomson Corporation.

Thomson and Star Logo are trademarks and Gale and Blackbirch Press are registered trademarks used herein under license.

For more information, contact
Blackbirch Press
27500 Drake Rd.
Farmington Hills, MI 48331-3535
Or you can visit our Internet site at http://www.gale.com

ALL RIGHTS RESERVED.
No part of this work covered by the copyright hereon may be reproduced or used in any form or by any means—graphic, electronic, or mechanical, including photocopying, recording, taping, Web distribution or information storage retrieval systems—without the written permission of the publisher.

Every effort has been made to trace the owners of copyrighted material.

Photo credits: Cover: all pictures Corel Corporation except for top center, © Royalty-Free/CORBIS; middle left © Digital Vision; middle right © Digital Stock; all pages © Discovery Communications, Inc. except for pages 4 © Royalty-Free/CORBIS; pages 8, 14 (bottom 3 images), 15, 24, 28, 36, 40 Corel Corporation; page 12 © Digital Vision; page 1, 20 © Digital Stock; page 39, National Archives

---

LIBRARY OF CONGRESS CATALOGING-IN-PUBLICATION DATA

Stinkers / John Woodward, book editor.
  p. cm. — (Planet's most extreme)
  Includes bibliographical references and index.
  ISBN 1-4103-0397-7 (hardcover : alk. paper) — ISBN 1-4103-0439-6 (paper cover : alk. paper)
  1. Smell—Juvenile literature. 2. Odors—Juvenile literature. 3. Glands, Odoriferous—Juvenile literature. 4. Physiology, Comparative—Juvenile literature. I. Woodward, John, 1958– II. Series.

QP458.S755 2005
612.8'6—dc22
                                                                                    2004018679

Printed in the United States of America
10 9 8 7 6 5 4 3 2 1

Animal Planet — THE MOST EXTREME

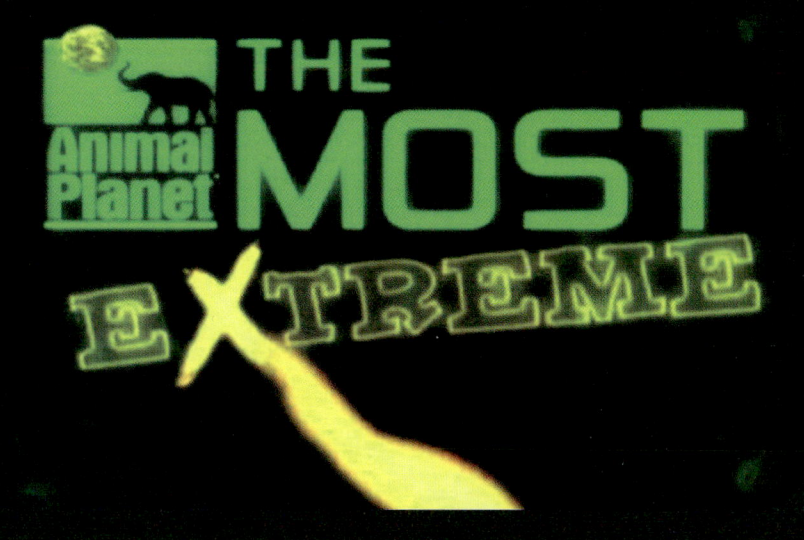

It's a dirty job, but someone's got to do it. We're going to count down the top ten most extreme stinkers in the animal kingdom, and compare them to people. Discover who's ahead by a nose when stink is taken to The Most Extreme.

10 The Dog

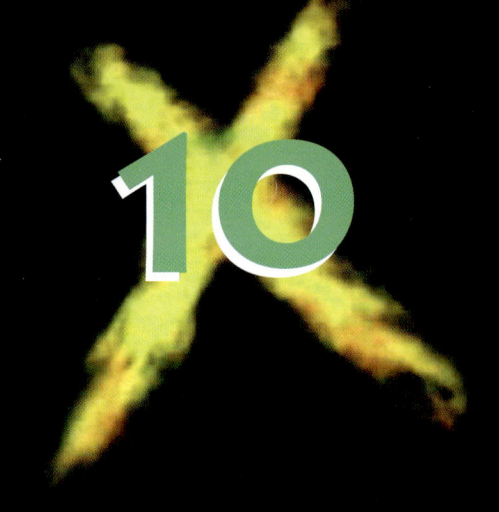

Walking into number ten in the countdown is an animal that can kick up a real stink. Dogs may be our best friends, but even the most devoted dog lover has to admit that Rover can smell revolting. They have a nasty habit of rolling in anything that stinks. And they just love sticking their noses into the nastiest places.

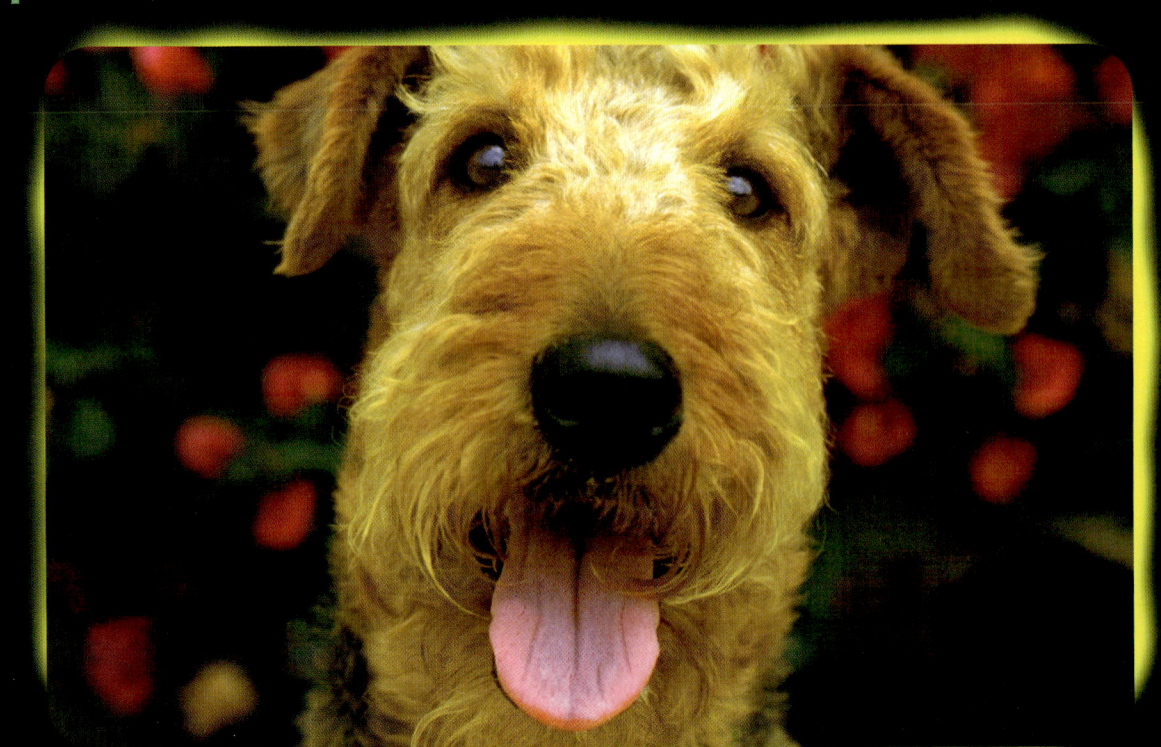

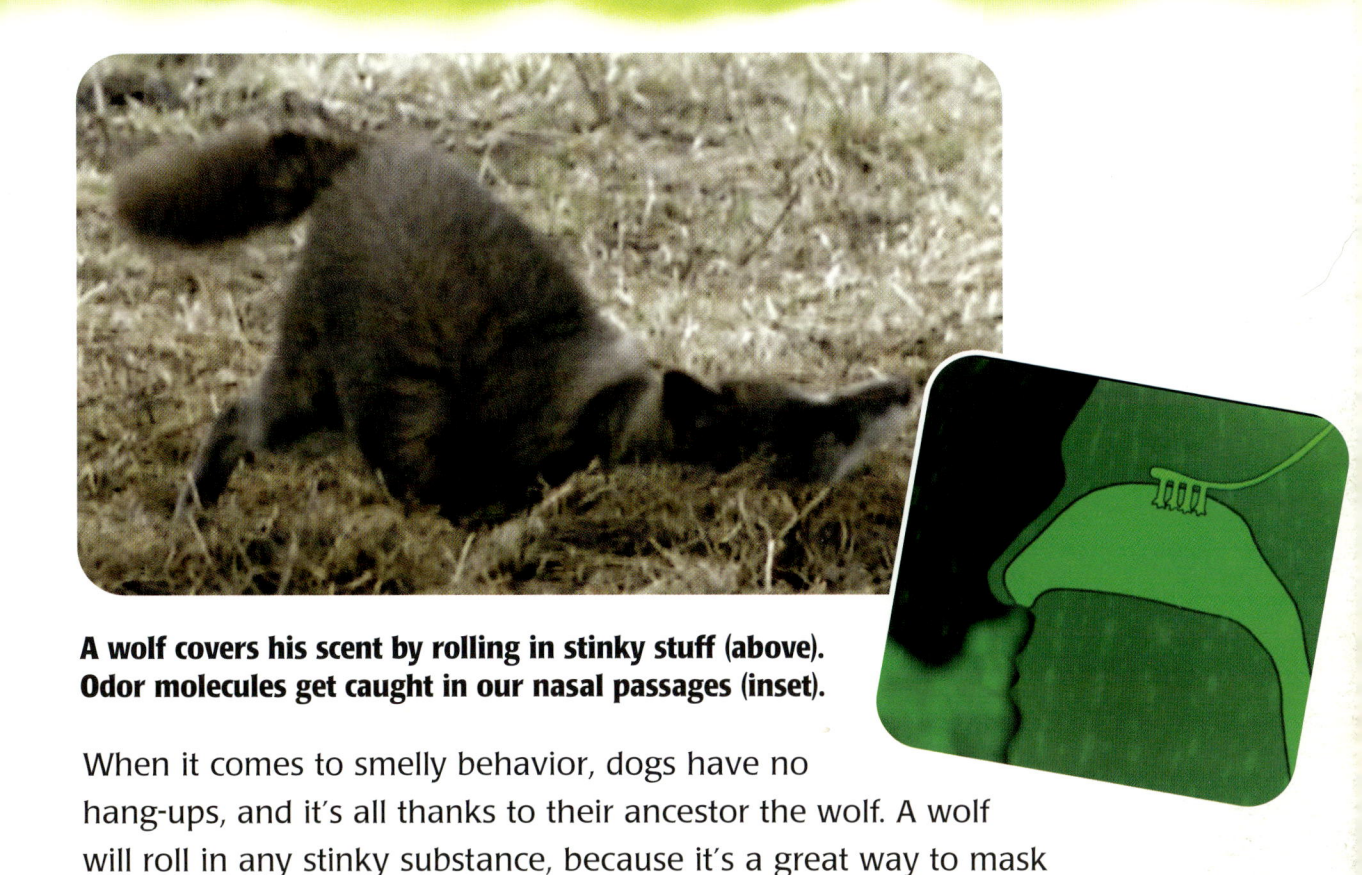

A wolf covers his scent by rolling in stinky stuff (above). Odor molecules get caught in our nasal passages (inset).

When it comes to smelly behavior, dogs have no hang-ups, and it's all thanks to their ancestor the wolf. A wolf will roll in any stinky substance, because it's a great way to mask its own scent so it can sneak up on dinner.

Today, the wolf's descendants still love to roll in anything that smells bad. And this gets right up our nose—literally. That's because when you encounter something that smells bad, molecules have evaporated off the noxious substance and floated through the air, up into your nose.

At the top of your nasal passages is a patch of special neurons about the size of a postage stamp. They're covered in hairlike projections that catch the odor molecules, and then trigger the nerves that tell your brain there's a smell in the air.

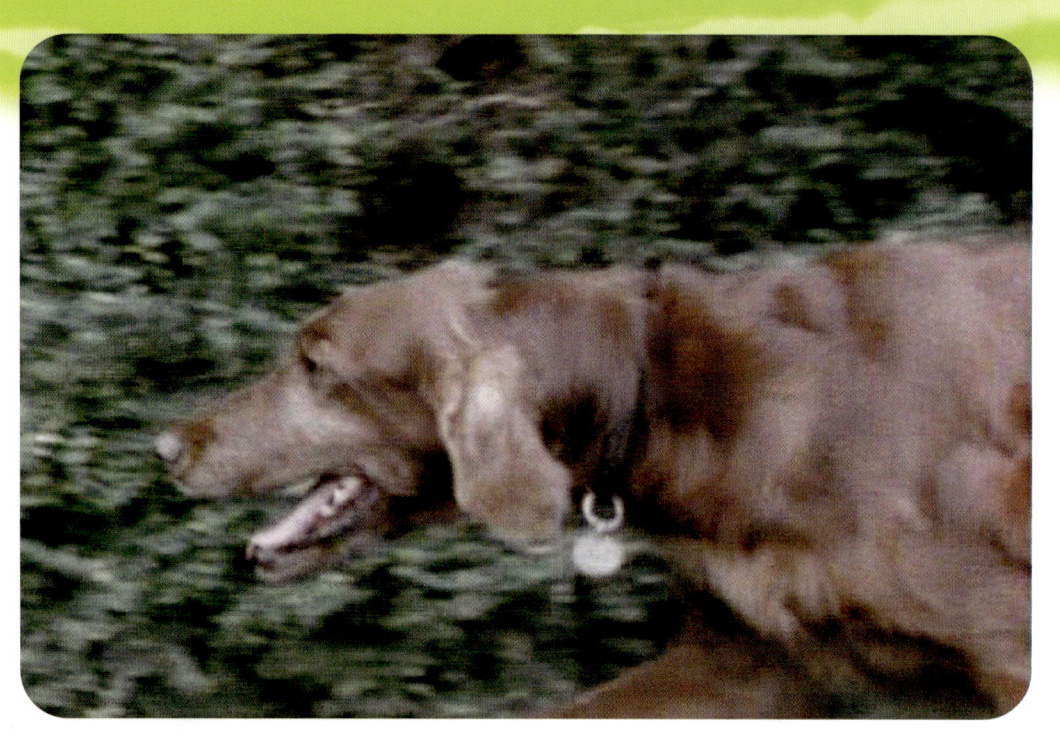

This dog chases after something he smells. A dog's sense of smell is far more sensitive than ours.

Our ability to sniff out stinks is very important, according to Pam Dalton, a researcher at the Monell Chemical Senses Center in Philadelphia:

> *Bad smells have significant potential to give us information about things we should avoid. We've been taught [this] from the time we're little children. If your mother took you into a public toilet, the first thing she said was, "Don't touch anything in here." We readily acquire the belief and the understanding that this is something that might hurt us.*

Imagine if we could smell as well as dogs! Their sense of smell is a million times more sensitive than ours. That's because their long snouts have more than ten times the area of smell receptor cells, and their wet noses act like Velcro, trapping scent molecules as they drift by.

Dogs often prefer to take a more direct route with their messages, attaching them to the local bulletin board—a tree. Both urine and droppings contain important scent signals that pass on information about the dog's sex, health, and even its mood. So the next time your pet dog leaves a message on your carpet—remember, it might just be trying to tell you how much it loves you.

These dogs leave scent messages for other dogs by urinating on trees.

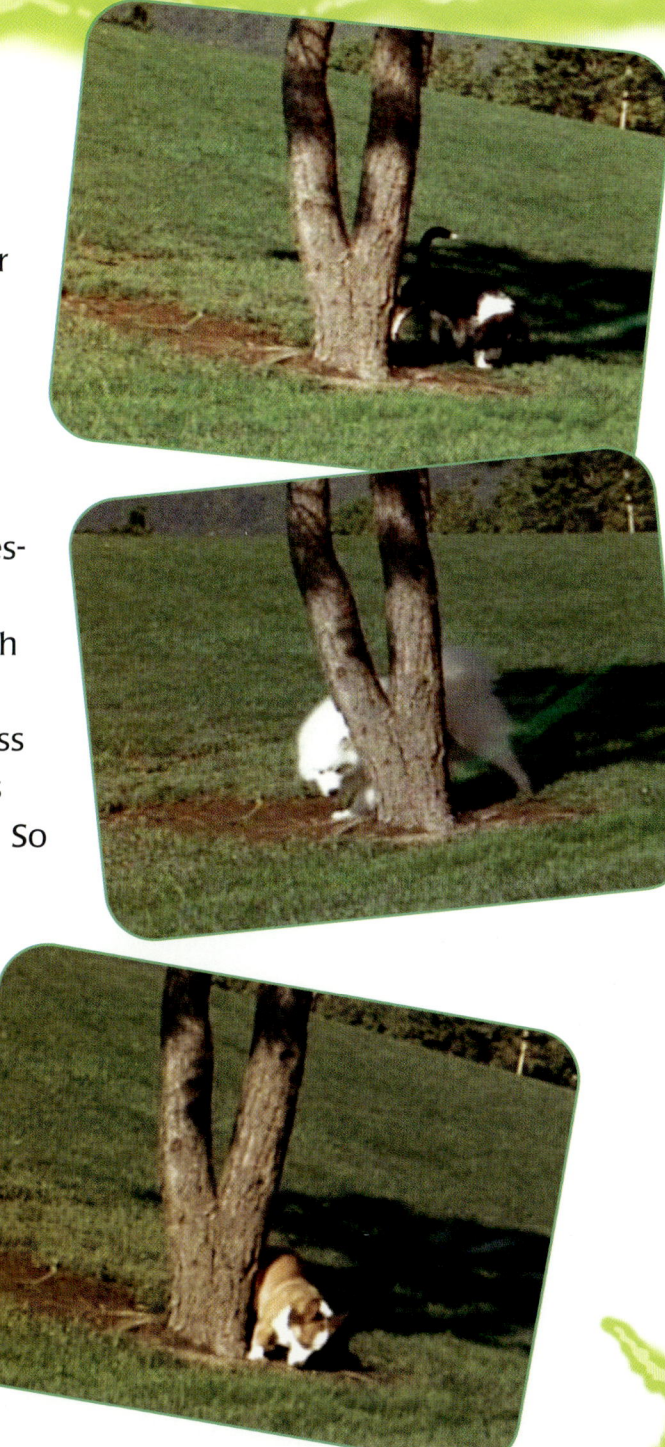

9

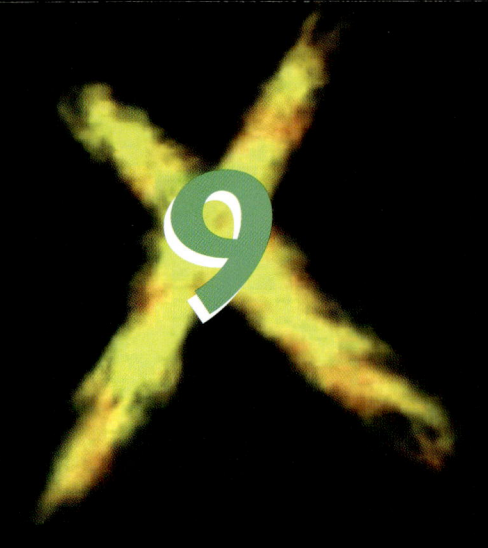

The Vulture

Every year thousands of visitors travel to Florida, attracted by the sea, sun, and scenery. But not all the tourists that flock here are welcome. Meet the vulture. It's firmly perched at number nine in the countdown because it has a truly disgusting way of keeping cool in the Florida sun.

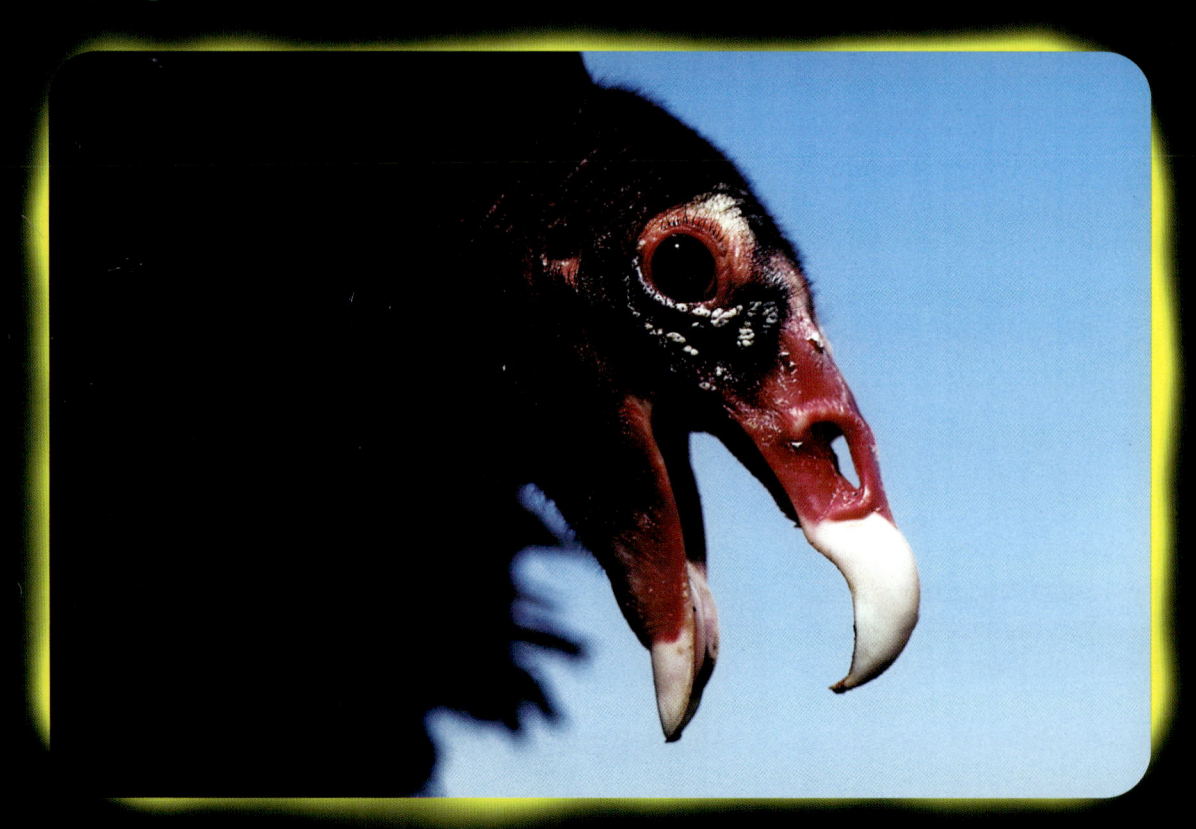

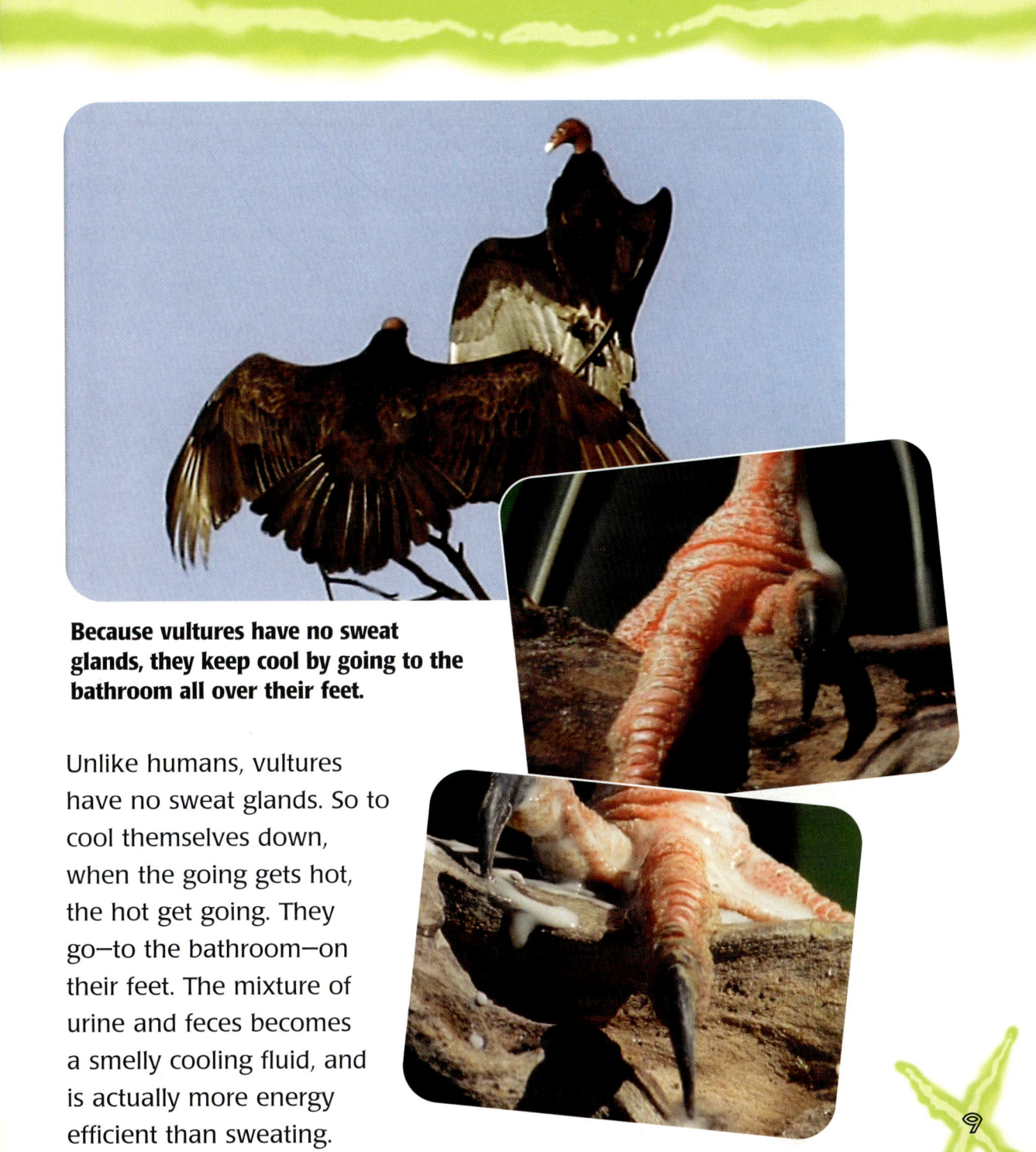

Because vultures have no sweat glands, they keep cool by going to the bathroom all over their feet.

Unlike humans, vultures have no sweat glands. So to cool themselves down, when the going gets hot, the hot get going. They go—to the bathroom—on their feet. The mixture of urine and feces becomes a smelly cooling fluid, and is actually more energy efficient than sweating.

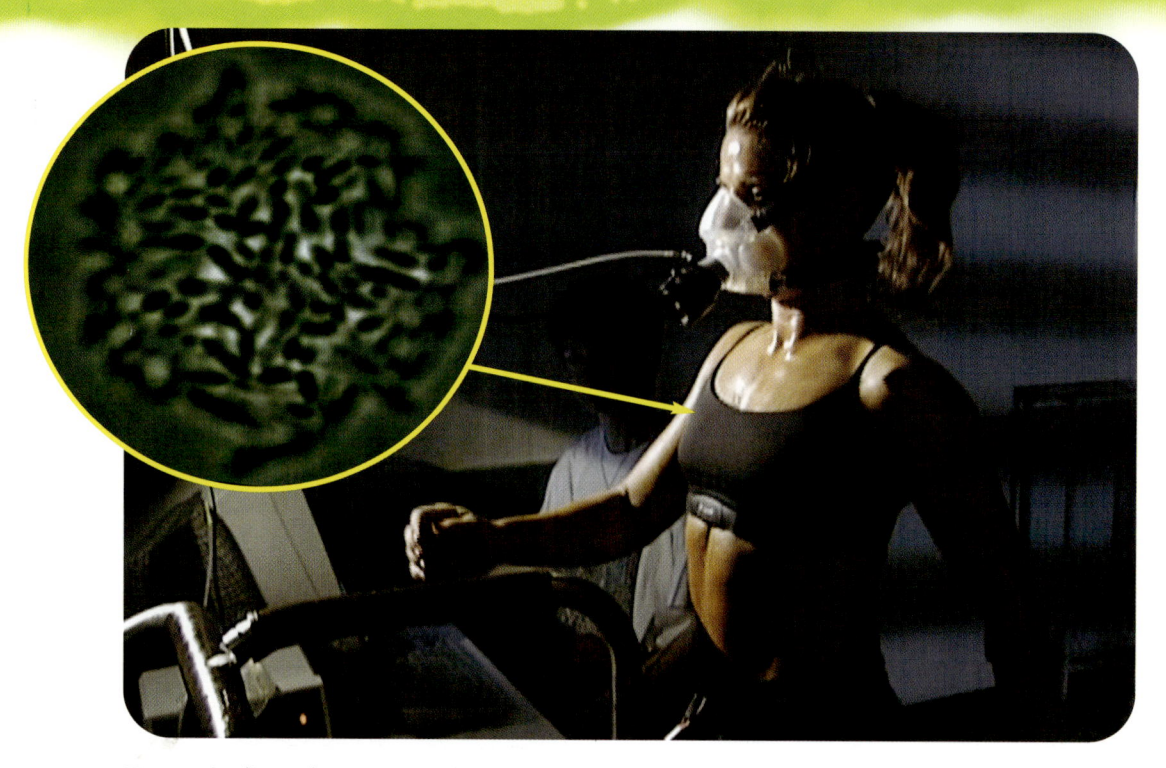

Bacteria (inset) are chowing down on the proteins and fatty acids under this woman's armpits as she sweats.

Thankfully, we have more than 2 million sweat glands in our skin that secrete mostly water, which cools our body as it evaporates. We may be disgusted by the vulture's behavior, but don't forget that our sweat glands can also produce some awful odors.

The sweat produced under our armpits contains proteins and fatty acids, which is the perfect food for bacteria. When the bacteria under our armpits excrete their waste products, we start to stink. That's why we only apply antiperspirants and deodorants to our armpits. It's also why 72 percent of American women say it is the one personal care product they couldn't live without.

Vultures have no need for antiperspirants, of course. They don't perspire, and it also seems that bacteria don't stand a chance against the vulture's novel approach to personal hygiene. Scientists have discovered that the high concentration of ammonia in vulture urine kills bacteria. So when they lunch at the local landfill, they don't care that their feet smell like a sewer!

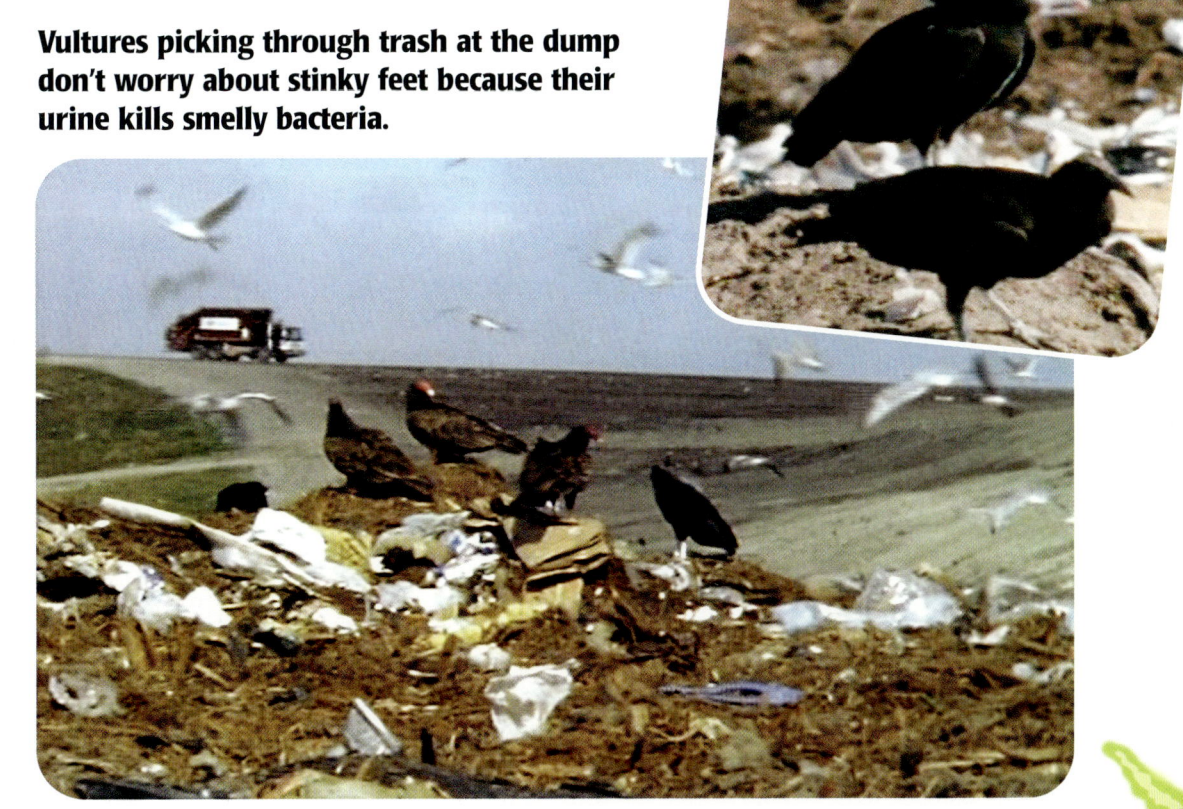

Vultures picking through trash at the dump don't worry about stinky feet because their urine kills smelly bacteria.

8 The **Hippopotamus**

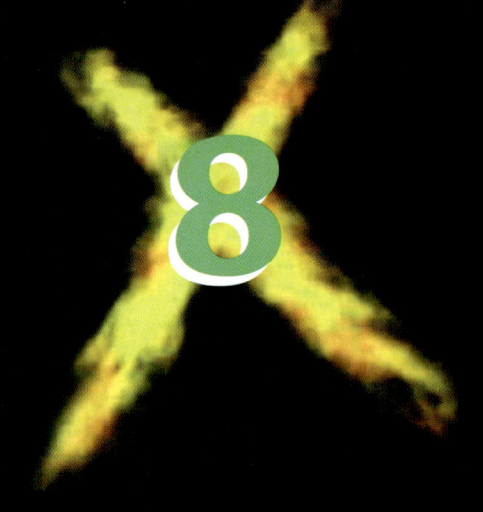

Travel down a river in Africa, and you stand a good chance of getting a noseful of number eight in our countdown of extreme stinkers. But it could be the last thing you ever smell. The hippopotamus is famous for its ability to detach your head from your shoulders with a single bite. But hippos have another way of overwhelming opposition, and it is truly disgusting.

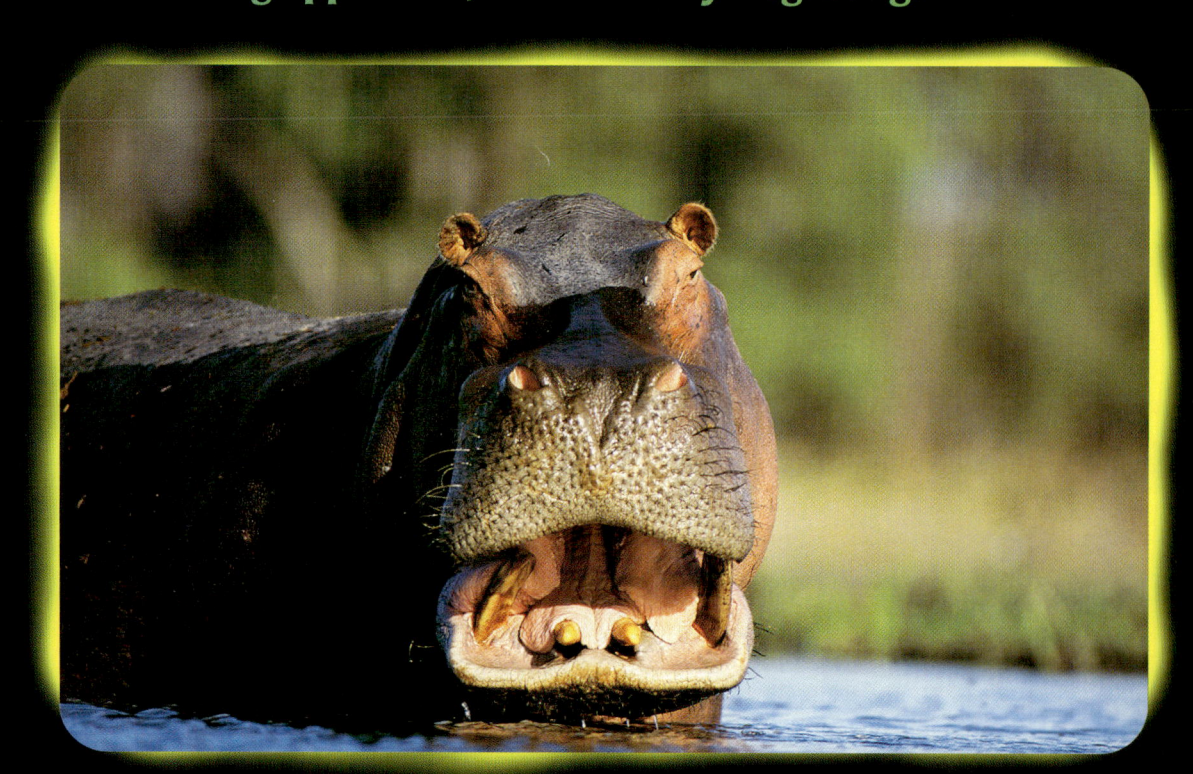

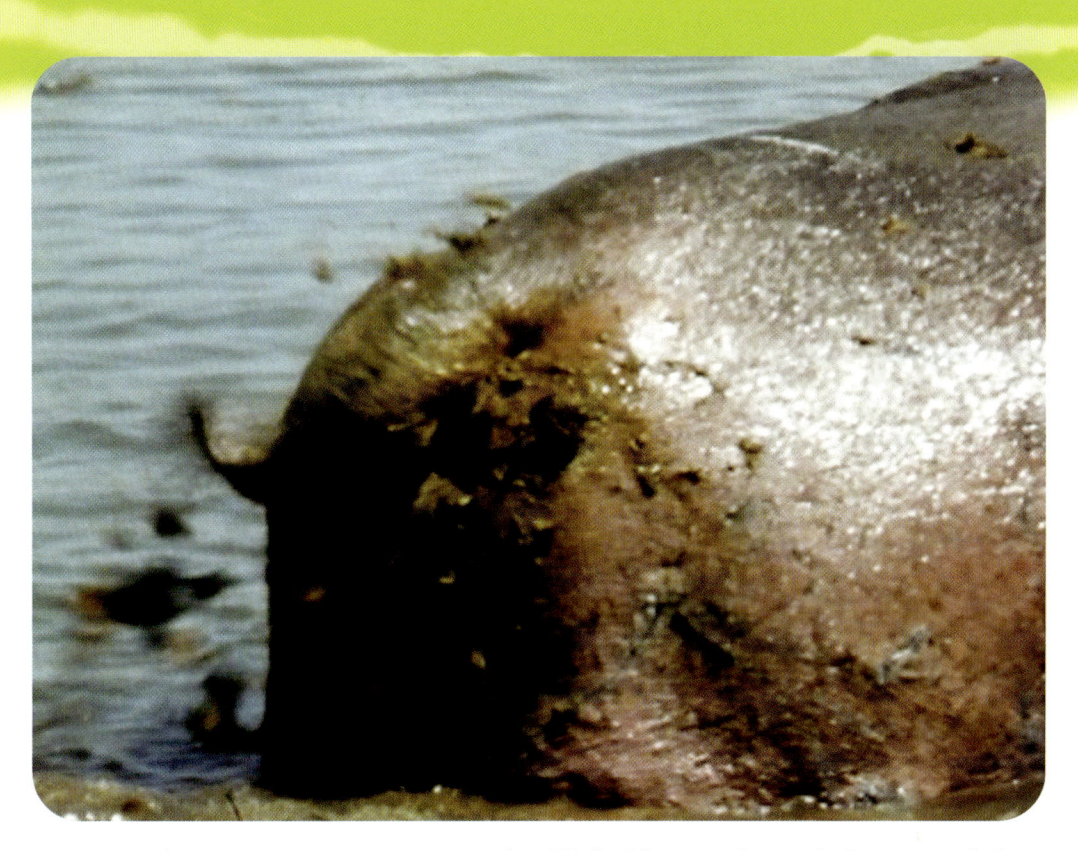

Here's a shower no one wants to take. Male hippos show their strength by showering dung all over.

The hippo's secret weapon is the result of its diet. Every night a hippo puts away over one hundred pounds of vegetation. As it travels through the hippo's massive intestines it starts fermenting, breaking down into a smelly soup. By the end of its journey the plant material has become a stinky green grenade ready to be thrown at any rival that gets too close for comfort.

Hippos are number eight in the countdown thanks to the dominance display known as "dung showering." Males show who's boss by twirling their tails like propellers to ensure the dung is sprayed all over.

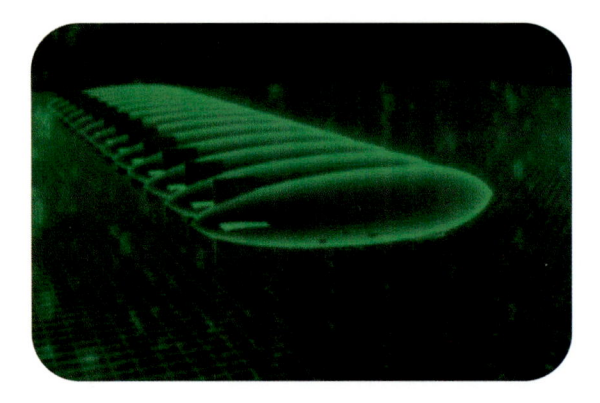

All the people in the world produce enough digestive gas every day to fill thirteen blimps!

Fortunately, people don't behave like hippos. But each day, the average human produces about 3.5 pints of digestive gases. If you could collect the gases produced by all the people in the world in one day, you'd have enough gas to fill thirteen blimps!

If you analyze the composition of our digestive gases, you'll find that the main ingredients are all odorless. The smell comes from the tiniest traces of sulfur. Onions and garlic are full of sulfur. Other foods, such as beans and cabbage, are broken down by bacteria that produce sulfurous stenches.

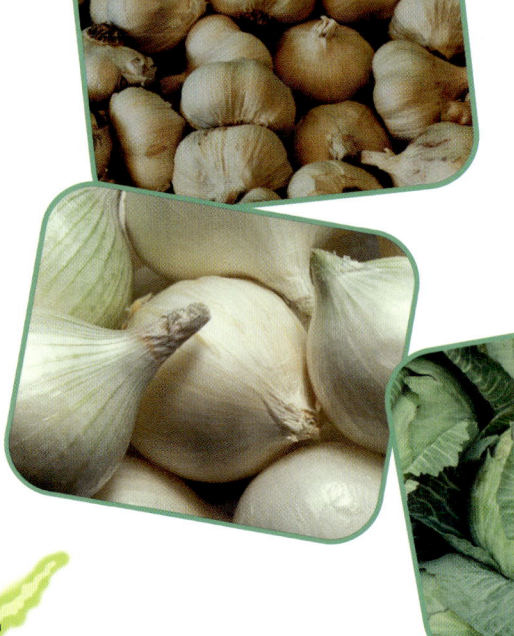

Foods such as garlic, onions, and cabbage produce a sulfur smell when digested.

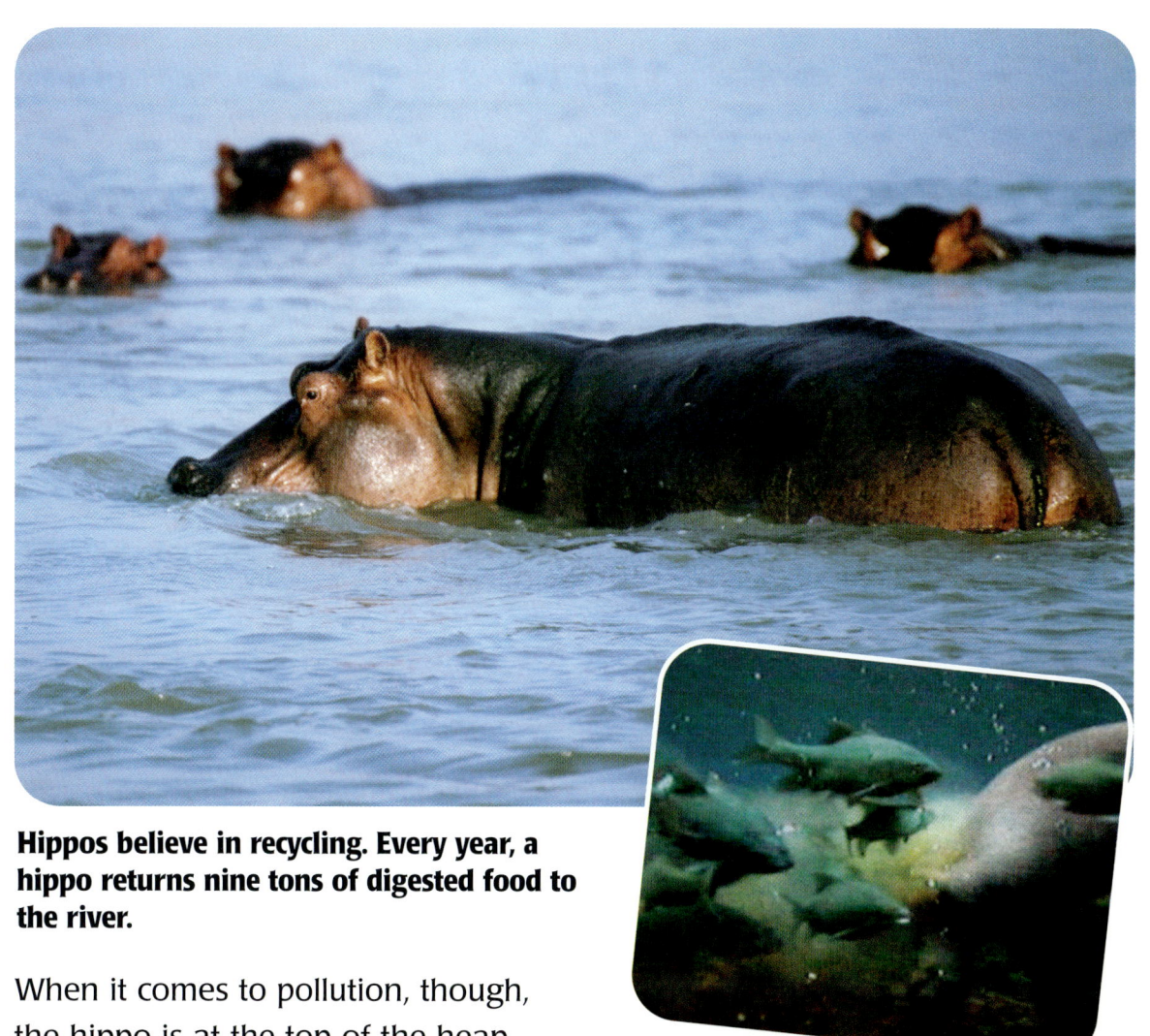

Hippos believe in recycling. Every year, a hippo returns nine tons of digested food to the river.

When it comes to pollution, though, the hippo is at the top of the heap. Every year a hippo deposits nine tons of predigested food back in the river.

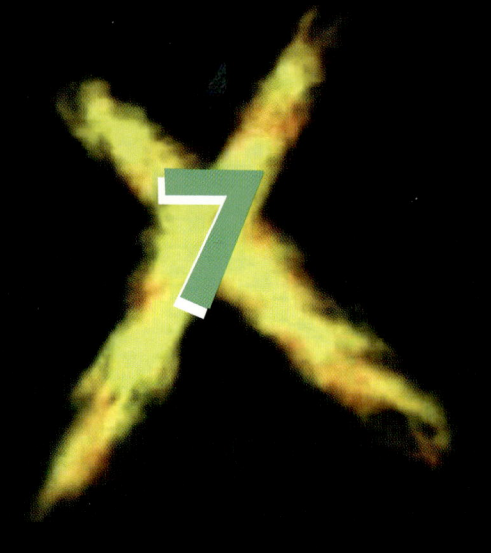

7
The Hooker's Sea Lion

To find the next contender in our countdown of extreme stinkers, we're traveling to the southern coast of New Zealand in search of a Hooker's sea lion, the rarest sea lion in the world. It's number seven in the countdown because it has extreme halitosis.

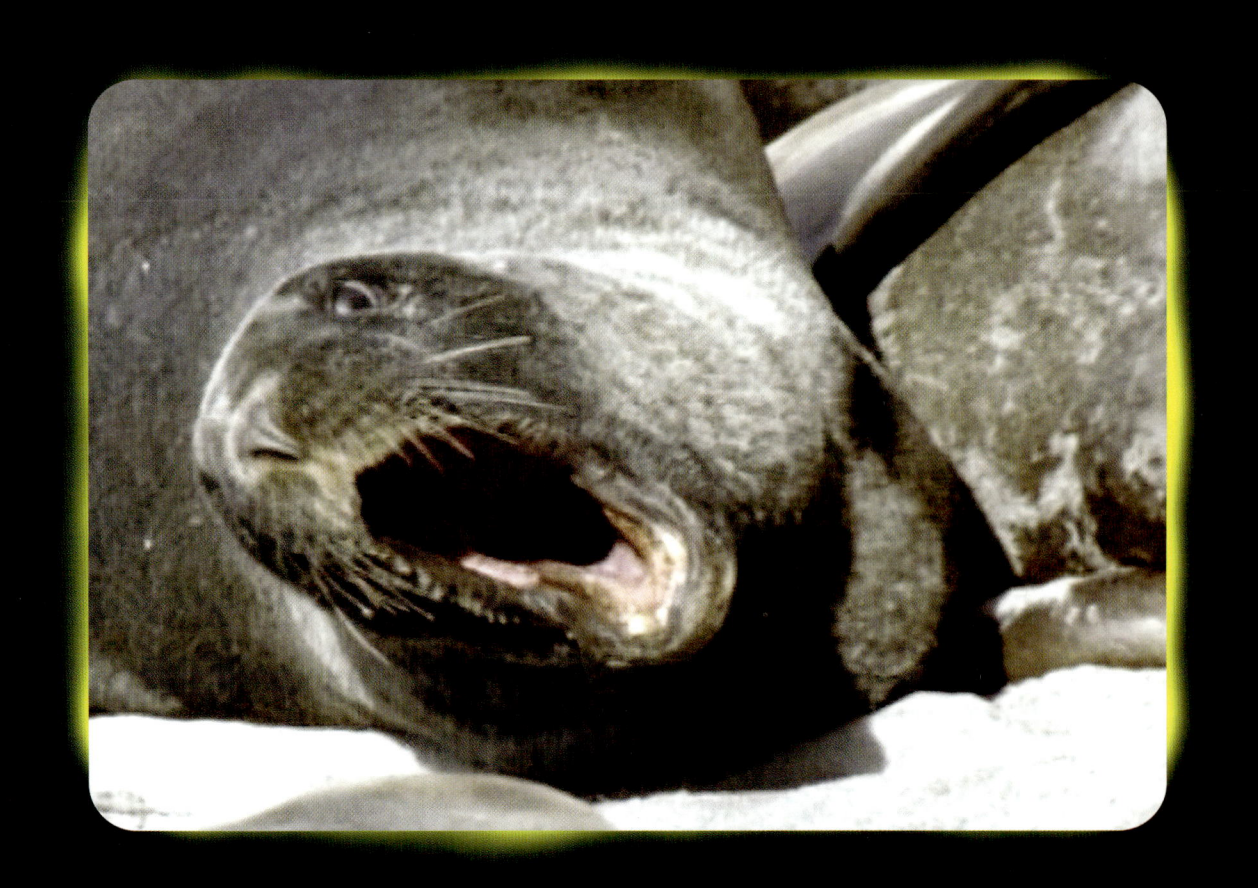

These Hooker's sea lions may be fighting over whose breath is stinkier, thanks to their all-fish diet.

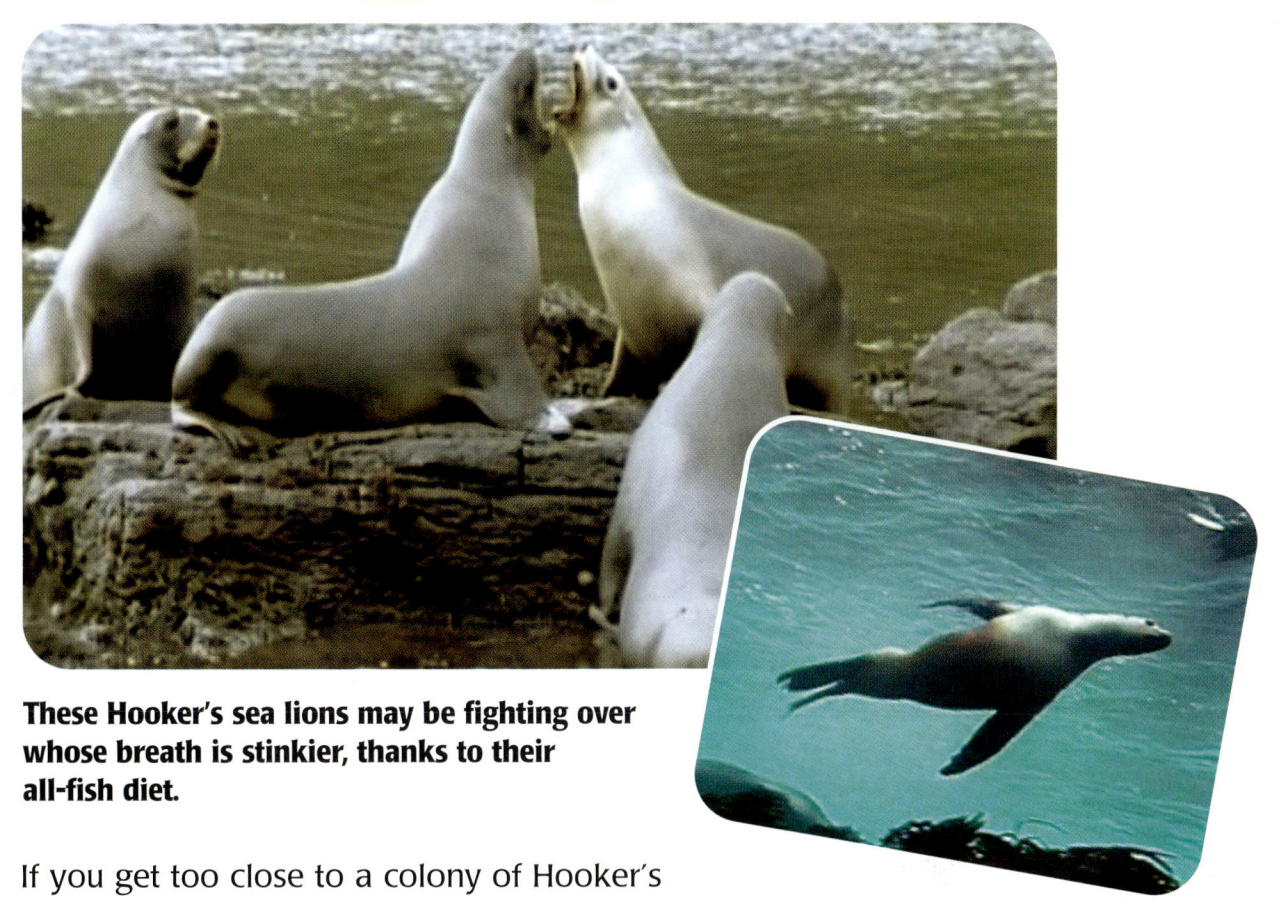

If you get too close to a colony of Hooker's sea lions, you'll quickly learn that they have spectacularly stinky breath. Their bad breath is nearly as deadly as their teeth, and it's all because of their diet. They like fish—lots of fish.

A sea lion will eat 60 pounds of fish every day on its underwater hunting trips. It's an incredible swimmer that can dive down more than 1,500 feet and hold its breath for an astonishing twelve minutes. Perhaps this is the best time to meet a Hooker's sea lion—when it's holding its breath!

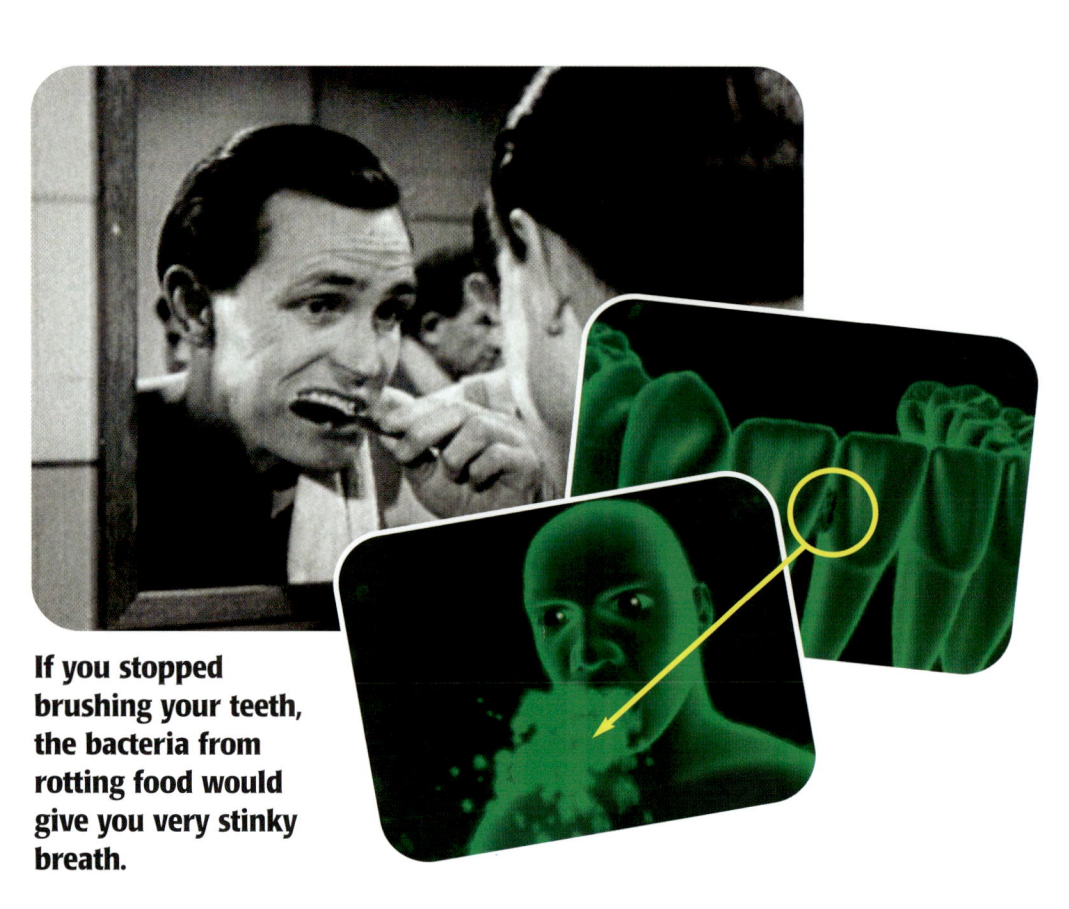

If you stopped brushing your teeth, the bacteria from rotting food would give you very stinky breath.

A sea lion can live for more than twenty years on its fishy diet. That's an awful long time without brushing or flossing! That's why this animal has such a foul mouth. Pieces of rotting food trapped in the teeth create bad breath for both sea lions and humans.

If you want breath like a Hooker's sea lion, simply stop brushing your teeth. Scraps of food will start decomposing in your mouth. Bacteria will flourish and start releasing the sulfurous gases that are the prime cause of bad breath.

An estimated 60 million Americans suffer from chronic halitosis, but not one of them can compare to the Hooker's sea lion. As if rotting fish breath wasn't bad enough, these extreme stinkers have found another way to add a foul flavor. Throwing up is the perfect way to get rid of those indigestible fishy leftovers and to add the aroma of vomit to already putrid breath.

Ever wonder how to get rid of undigested fish? A Hooker's sea lion just vomits it back up.

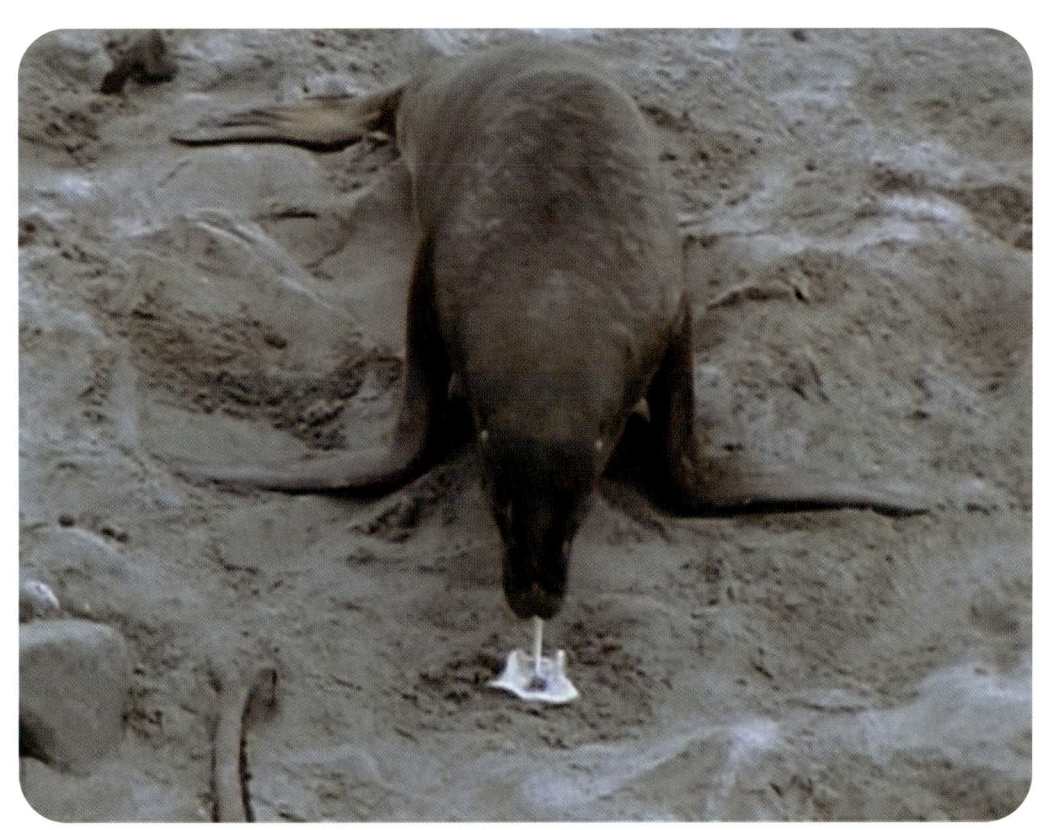

6 The Hyena

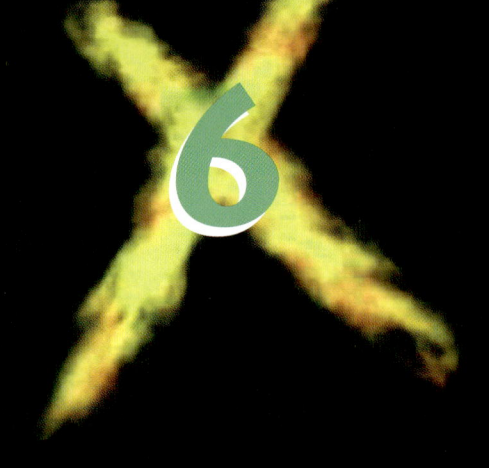

When we're in the wilderness, it's easy to get lost. But our next contender never has to ask directions because it's surrounded by stinky signposts. The plains of Africa are home to number six in the countdown: the spotted hyena. The savanna may look deserted to us, but the average hyena is hardly ever more than 150 feet from its foul-smelling scent markers.

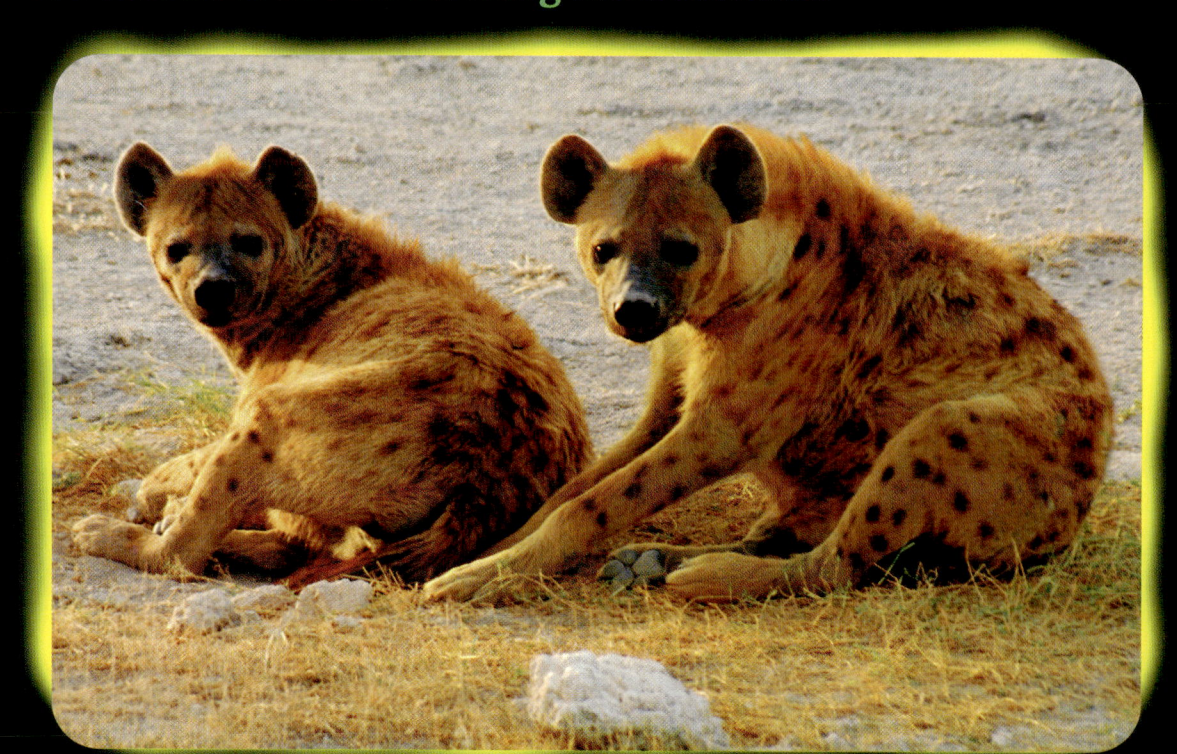

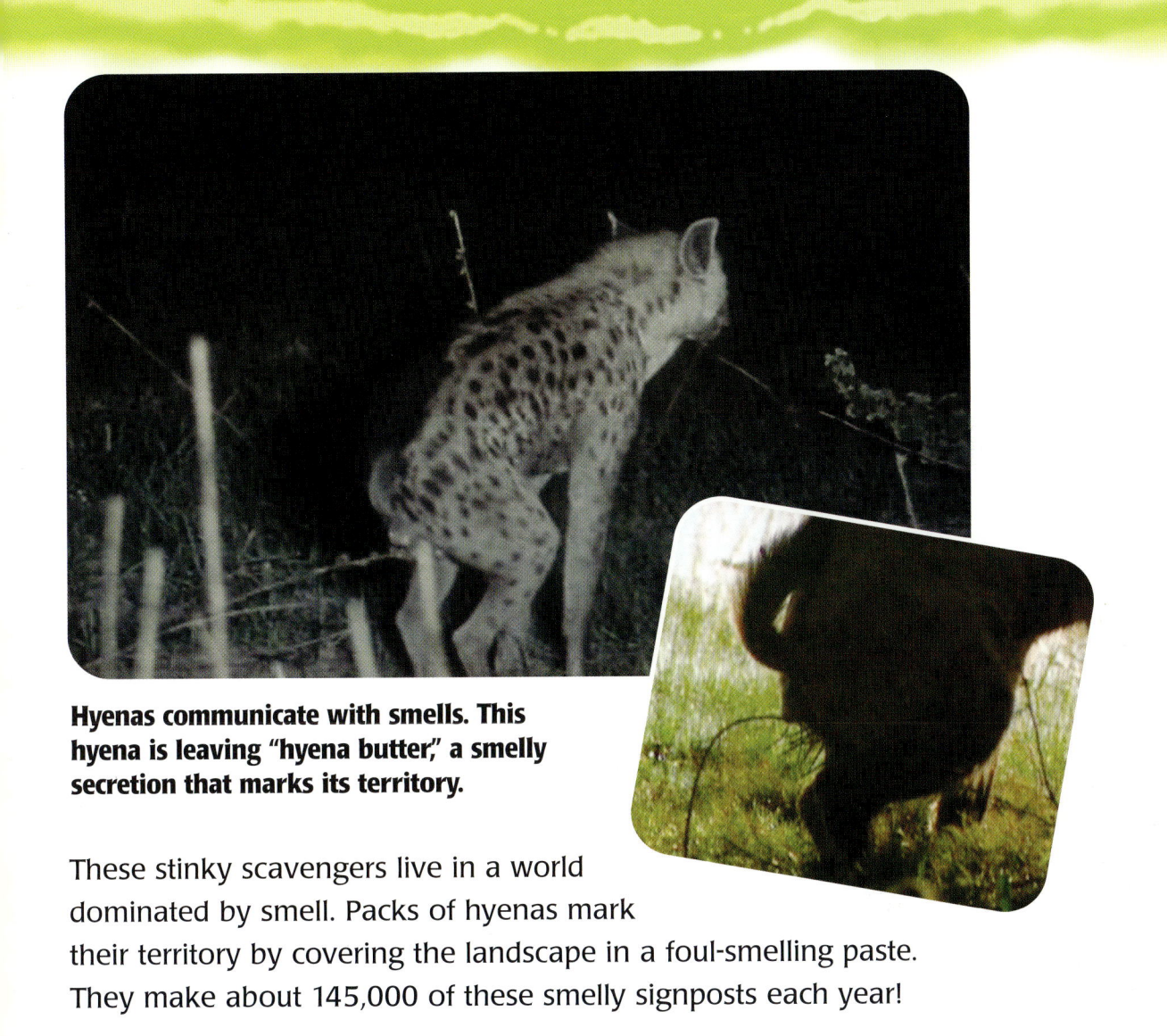

Hyenas communicate with smells. This hyena is leaving "hyena butter," a smelly secretion that marks its territory.

These stinky scavengers live in a world dominated by smell. Packs of hyenas mark their territory by covering the landscape in a foul-smelling paste. They make about 145,000 of these smelly signposts each year!

At night hyenas really get down to business—smelly business. Hyenas are number six in the countdown because they produce the stinky paste known as "hyena butter." Each pasting is so potent that it'll continue to reek for an amazing thirty days, broadcasting information about the pack to any hyena that strays into their territory. But hyenas aren't the only creatures that use smell to communicate.

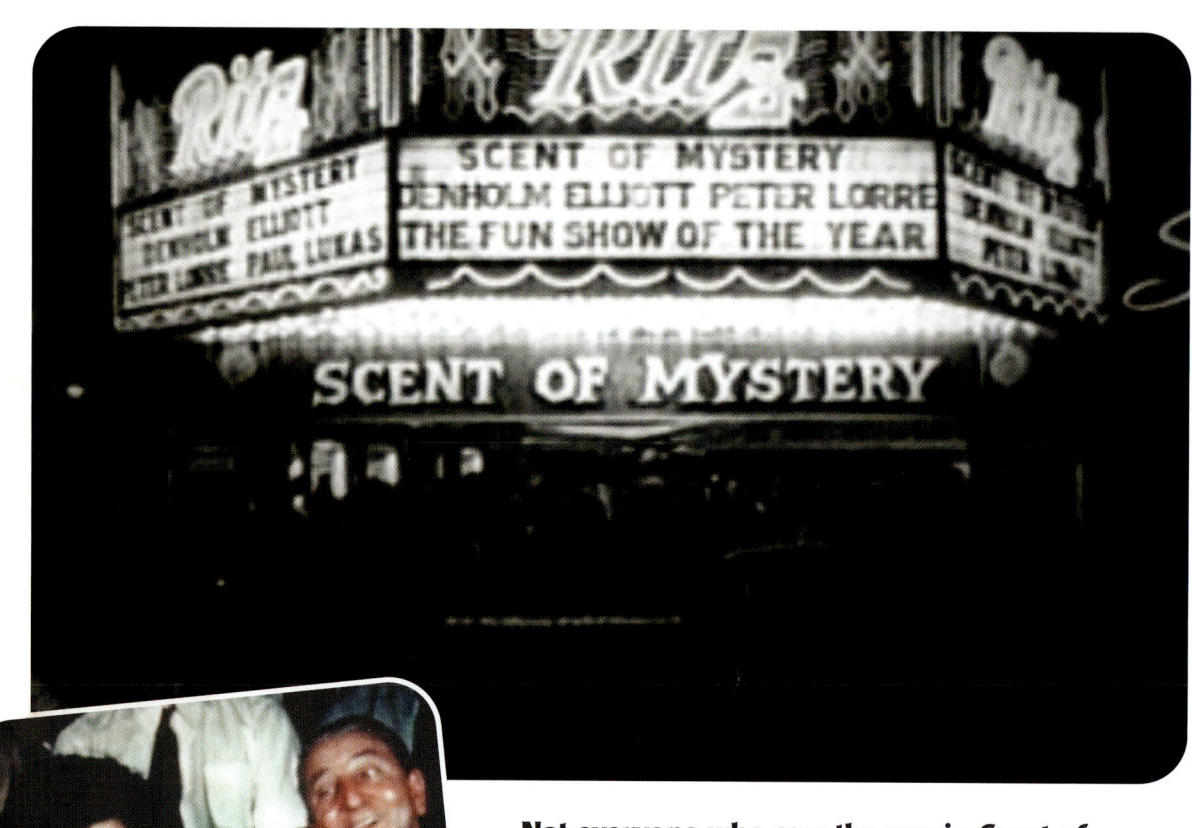

Not everyone who saw the movie *Scent of Mystery* in Smell-O-Vision enjoyed the smells in the theater!

In 1960, Hollywood saw the premiere of the *Scent of Mystery*, which was filmed in glorious "Smell-O-Vision." The theater had been specially modified to pump smells over the audience. The idea was that people would experience the smells of a barbecue, for example, at the same time as the action was sizzling on-screen.

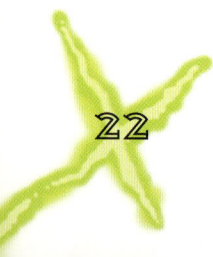

Unfortunately, Smell-O-Vision had problems. Audiences received the smells out of synch and, between showings, it was difficult to flush the scents out of the theaters. As word spread, the idea was abandoned.

Unlike human audiences, hyenas would have loved Smell-O-Vision. Although all that hyena butter probably wouldn't taste very good on the popcorn.

These hyenas are busy squeezing out hyena butter everywhere. They would have loved Smell-O-Vision.

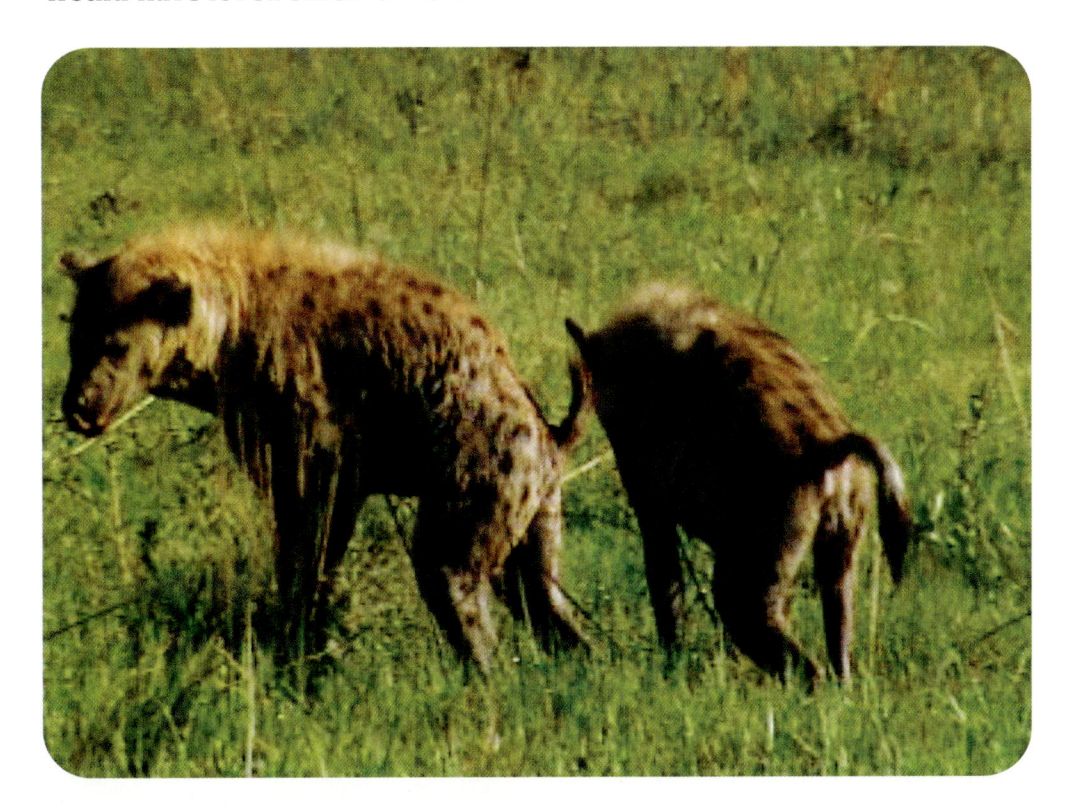

5 The Musk Ox

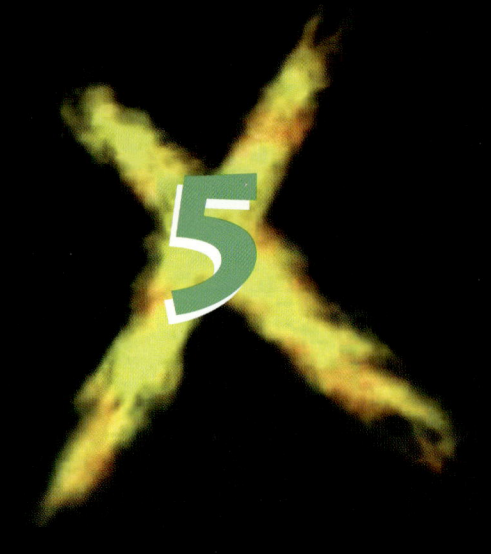

Before the development of a synthetic replacement, most perfumes contained a foul-smelling extract from a musk deer's anal glands. Perfume manufacturers had to dilute it, because in its natural state, real musk really stinks! You'd think that the biggest producer of musk in the world would be the animal that's coming in at number five in the countdown: the musk ox. But, actually, it's not.

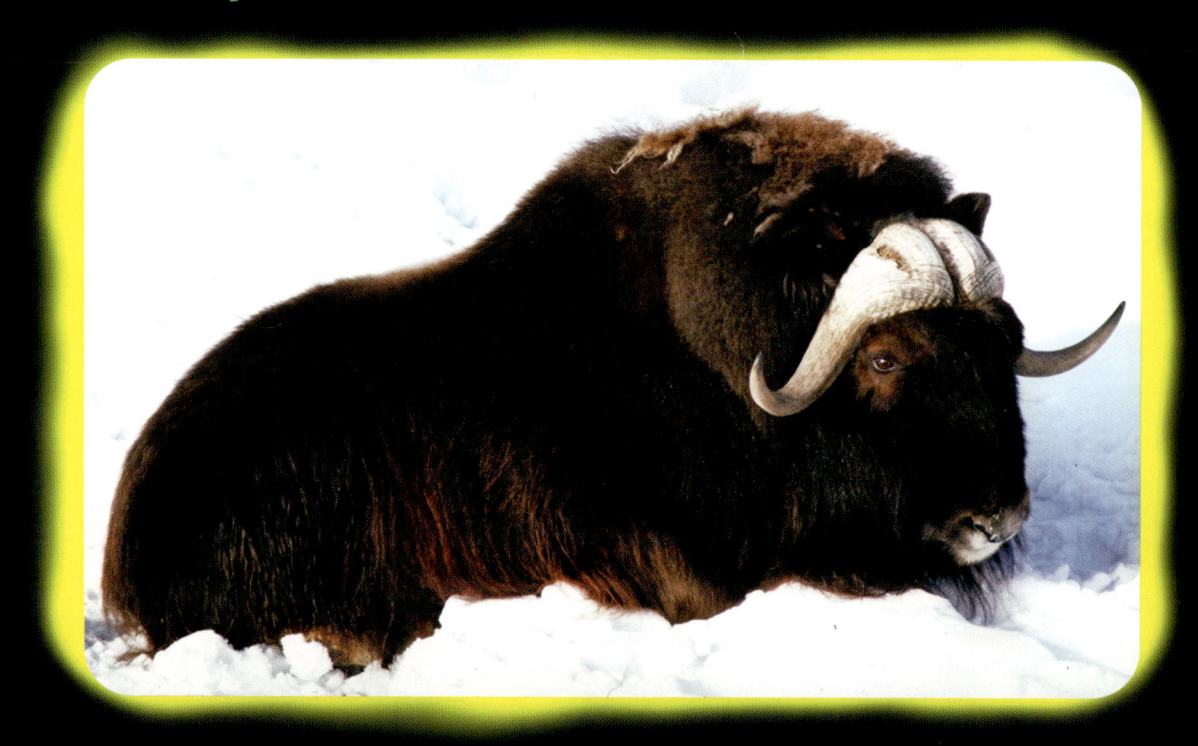

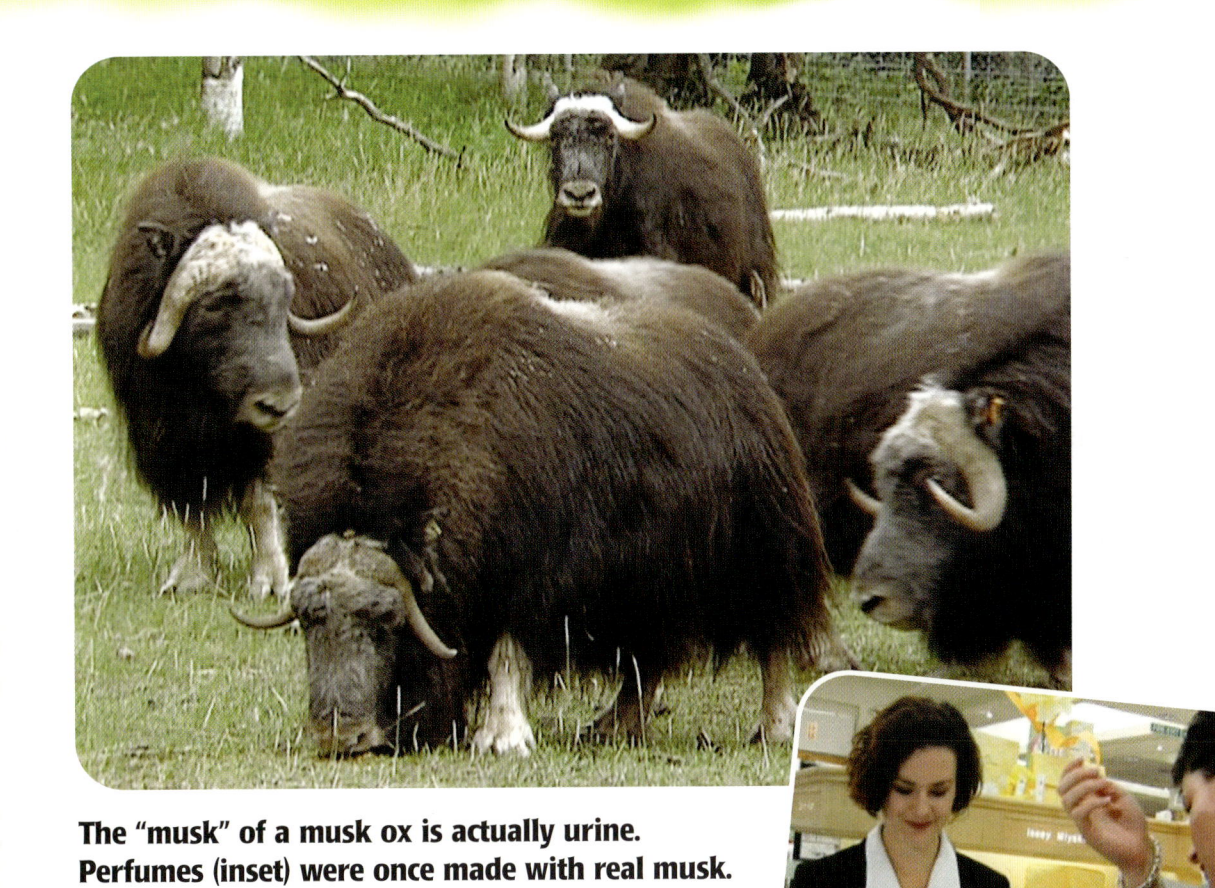

The "musk" of a musk ox is actually urine. Perfumes (inset) were once made with real musk.

If musk smells so bad, why has it been used in perfumes? For centuries, tiny amounts of musk were used as a fixative to make the other fragrances in the perfume stronger.

Surprisingly, the musk ox doesn't make musk and isn't an ox. This shaggy creature is more closely related to a sheep than an ox, and it doesn't have musk glands. Musk ox "musk" is actually urine. Try putting that in your perfume!

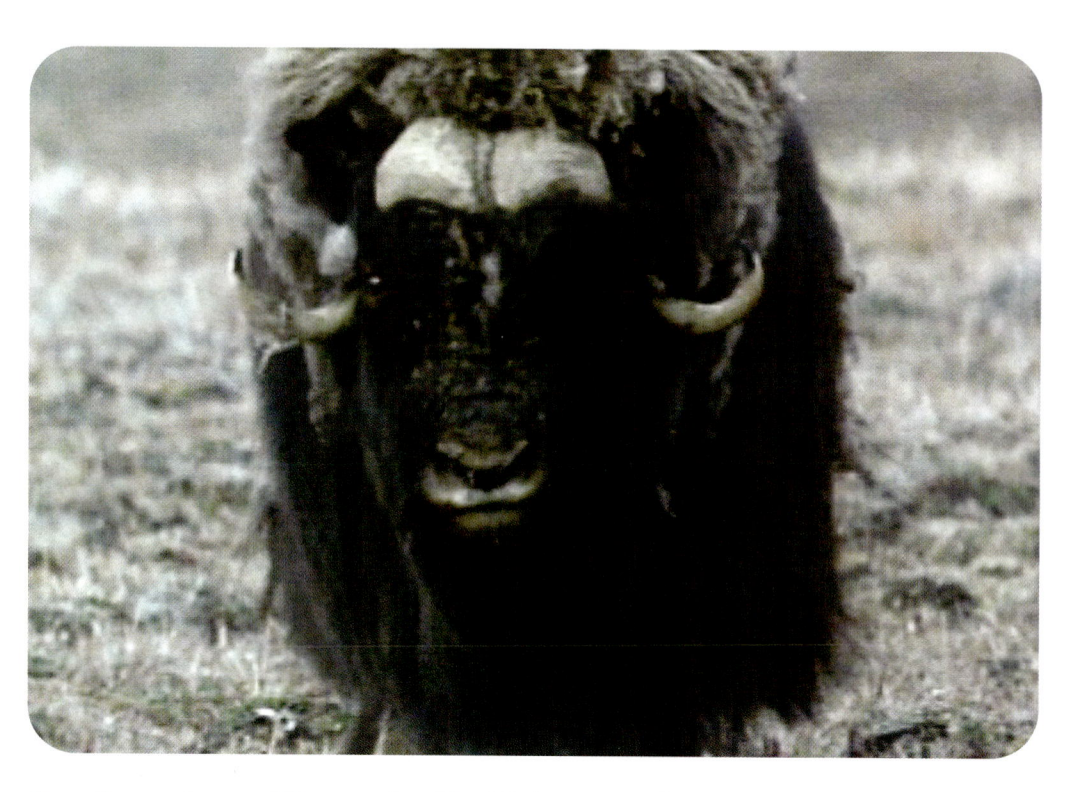

A male musk ox will spray itself with its very stinky urine to scare off other males.

A male musk ox liberally douses itself with urine to see who can make the biggest stink. Stand downwind and the musky smell is strong enough to make your eyes water! If smell alone isn't enough to scare off the competition, they butt heads. You would need to be knocked in the head to think that musk smells good!

The dawn of disco ushered in a new era for purified musk oil. Some thought the earthy animal odor was attractive. That's why dance floors in the seventies were saturated with the smell. However, not even the most ardent disco king would consider wearing a perfume of musk ox urine.

During the disco days of the 1970s, wearing musk oil (inset) as perfume on the dance floor was all the rage.

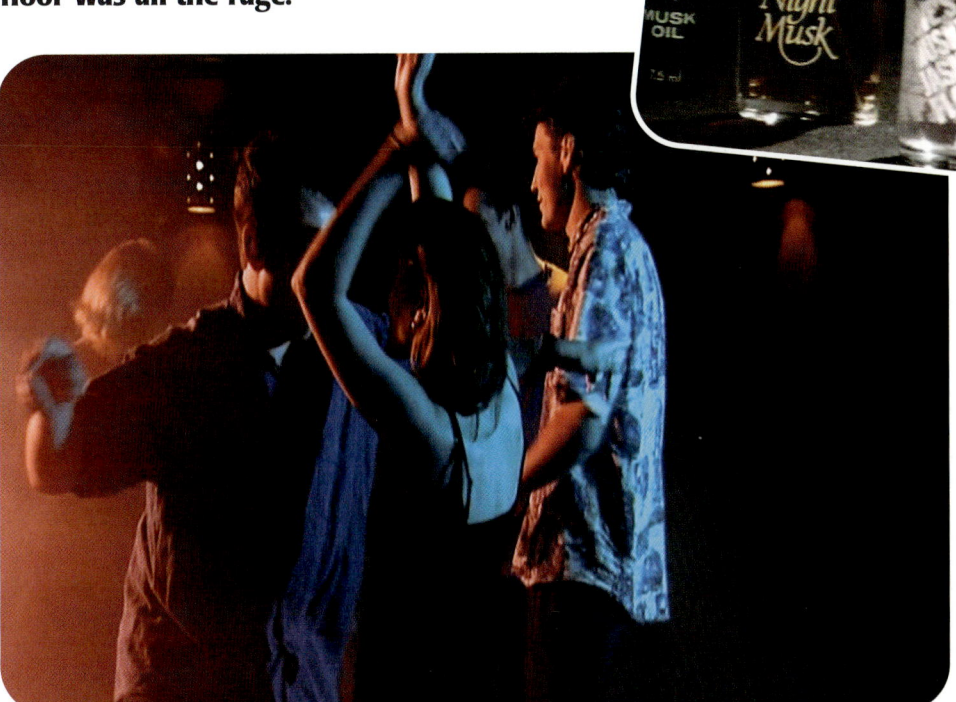

4

The Bull Elephant

Our next contender is the biggest stinker on the planet. The bull elephant is number four in the countdown because for one month every year, it really stinks.

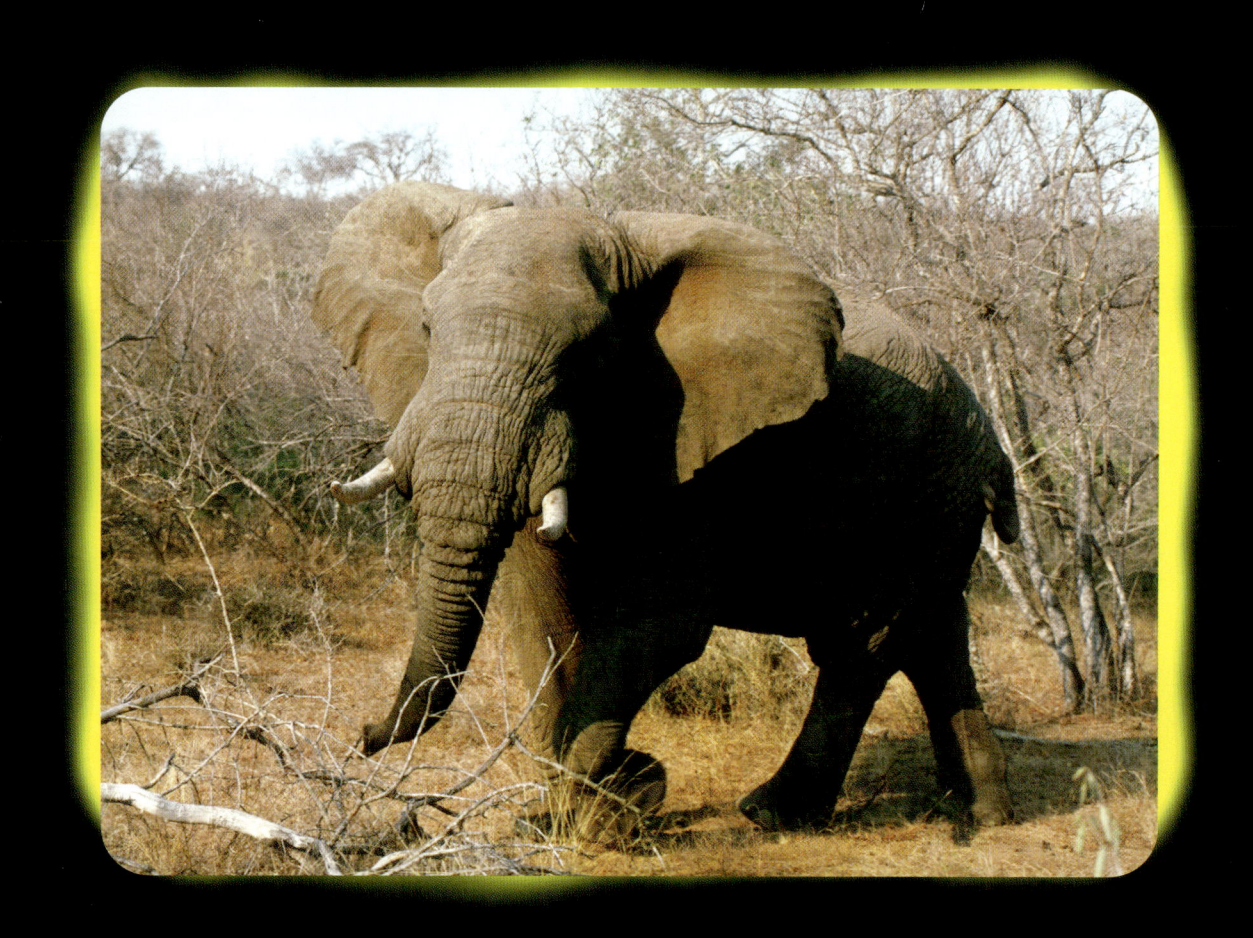

The rancid smell secreted by a bull elephant is called musth. Female elephants find musth quite attractive.

Take a close look at a bull's head and you can see a small gland between the eye and ear. When the bull's testosterone level skyrockets, this gland dribbles out a rancid-smelling secretion called musth. In Hindi, musth means "intoxicated," because bull elephants in musth are aggressive and smell really bad.

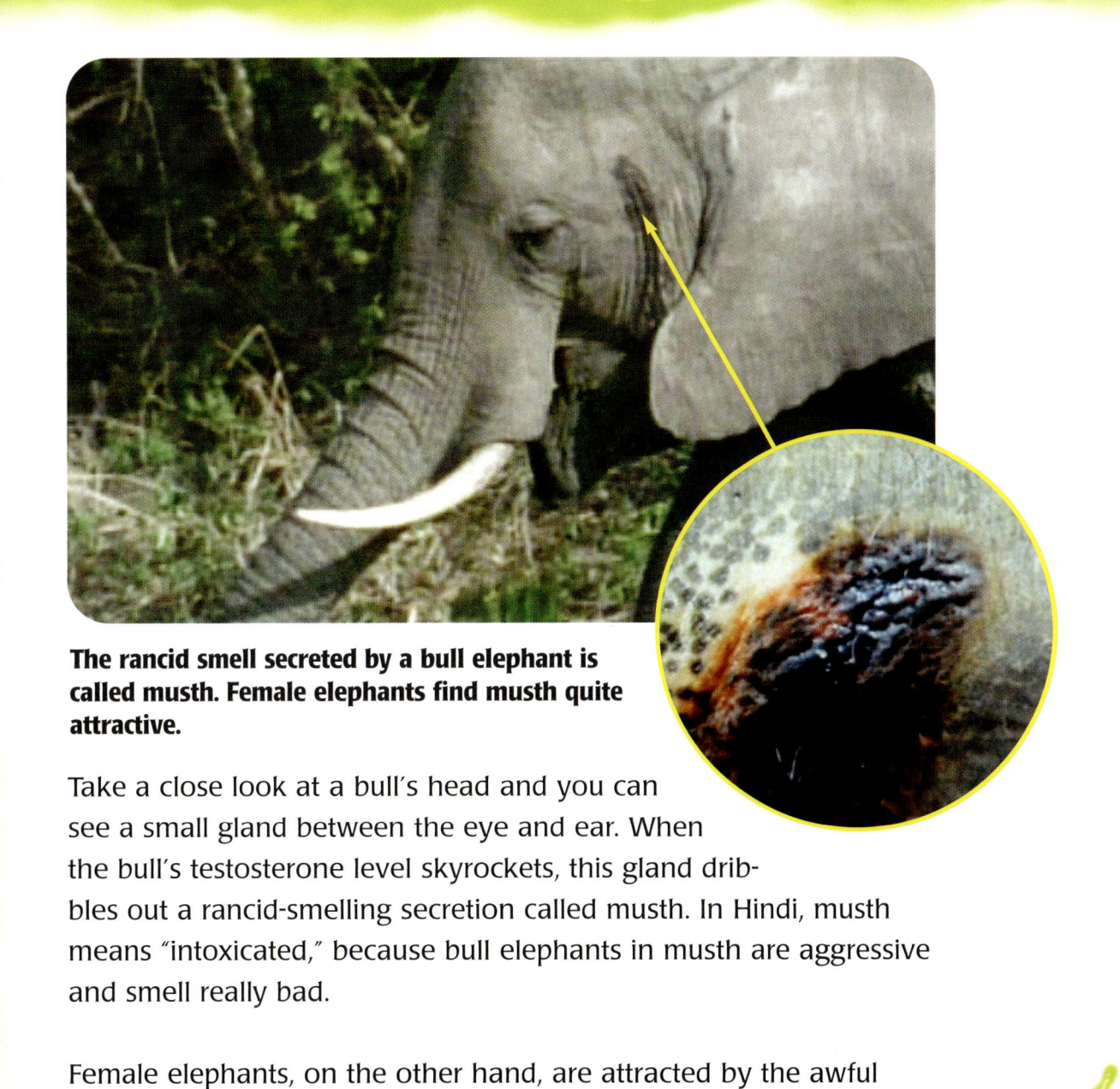

Female elephants, on the other hand, are attracted by the awful odor. They interpret the pungent smell as a sign of a healthy bull.

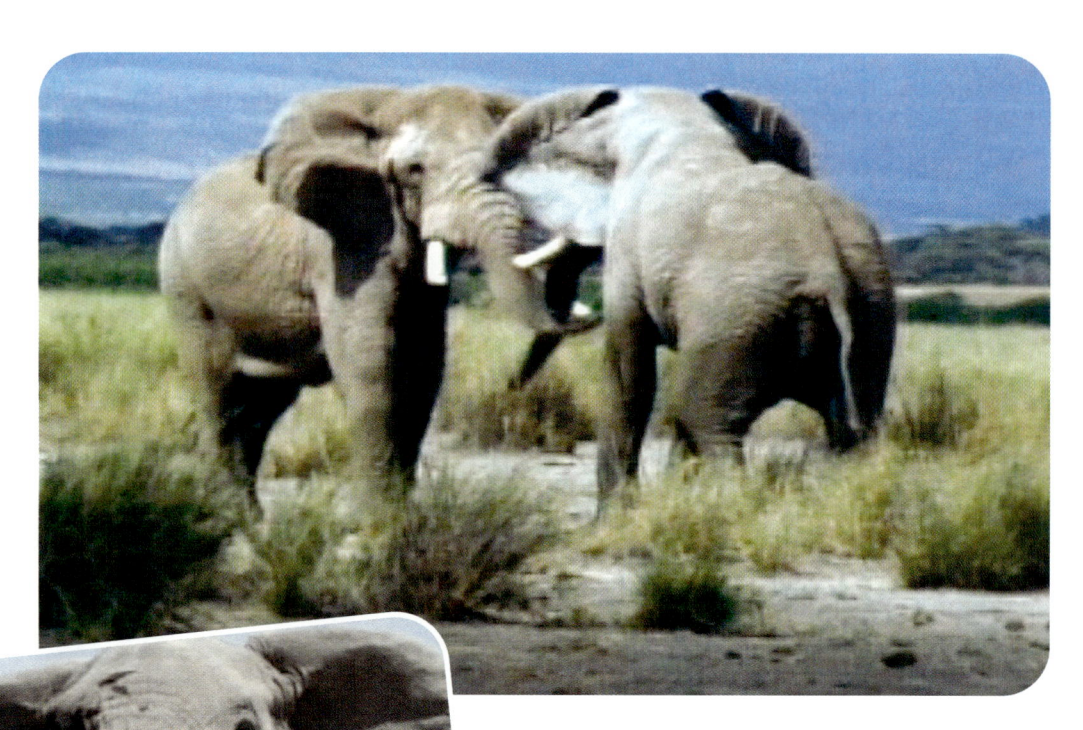

Bull elephants in musth can fight to the death over mating rights to a female.

Other males are less impressed with the odor. Elephants in musth have been known to kill each other in the fight for the right to mate.

All humans secrete pheromones as a part of their natural body odor. These chemicals send subtle messages that affect our behavior. The less we wash, the more pheromones we release.

Dr. Winnifred Cutler of the Athena Institute in Pennsylvania is an expert when it comes to invisible attractants. As part of a study, researchers laced women's favorite perfume with either Dr. Cutler's synthetic pheromone or a placebo. At the end of the study, the group wearing the synthetic pheromone reported a more than 70 percent increase in their popularity with the opposite sex! Dr. Cutler has used her research to commercially develop chemical extracts of human pheromones for both women and men.

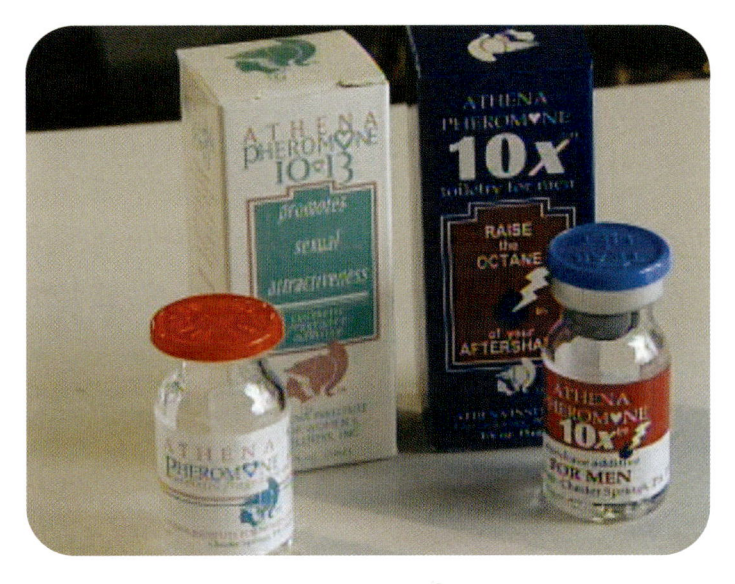

Some people wear synthetic pheromones to make themselves more attractive to the opposite sex.

Elephant perfume has been described as smelling like a thousand goats in a pen. No wonder adolescent male elephants are kicked out of the herd as soon as they start to stink!

3 The Millipede

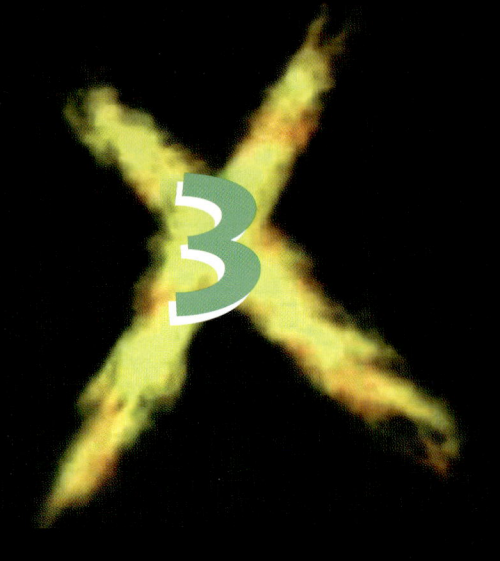

The next contender in our countdown of extreme stinkers can be found in forests around the world. Most people think of millipedes as harmless. But if they get threatened, they can create such a stink that even the hungriest hunter would turn up its nose at them.

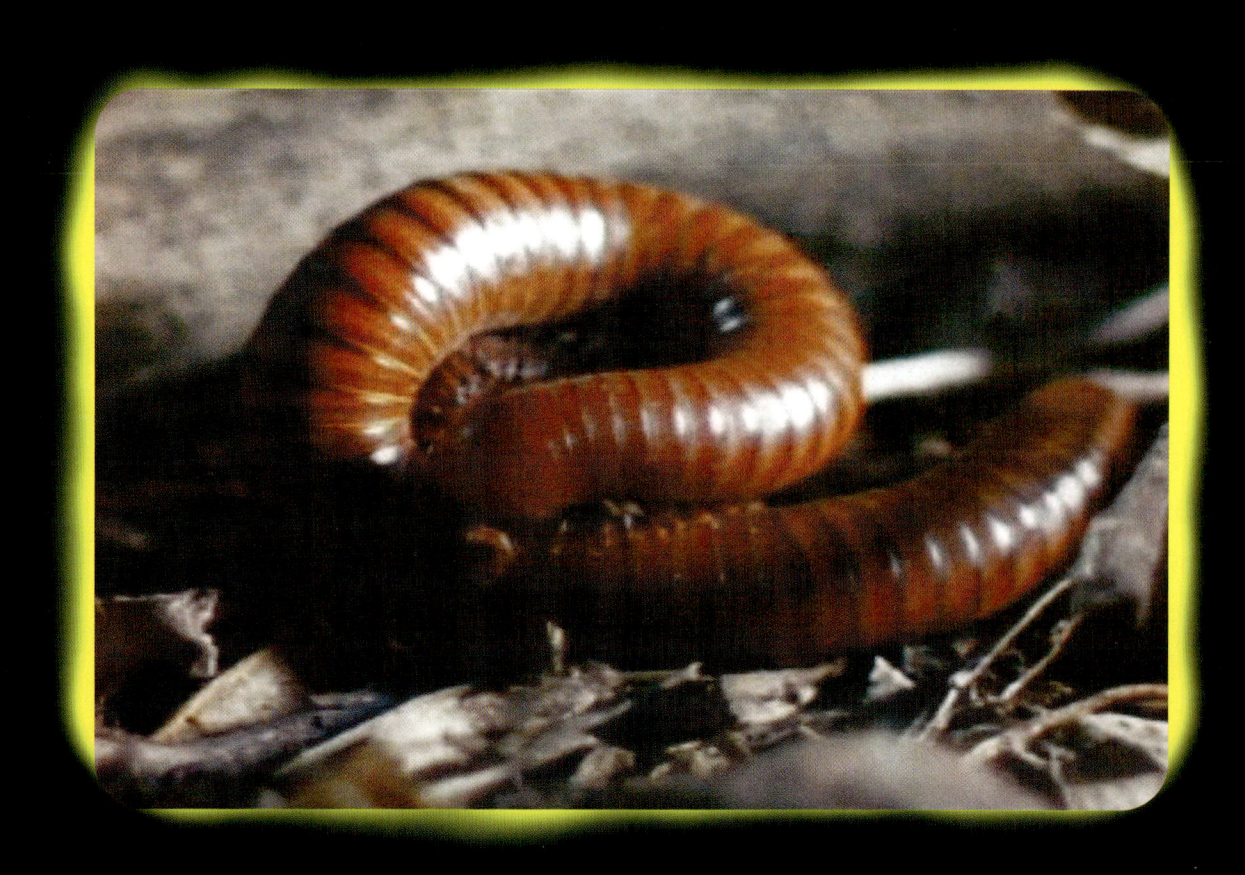

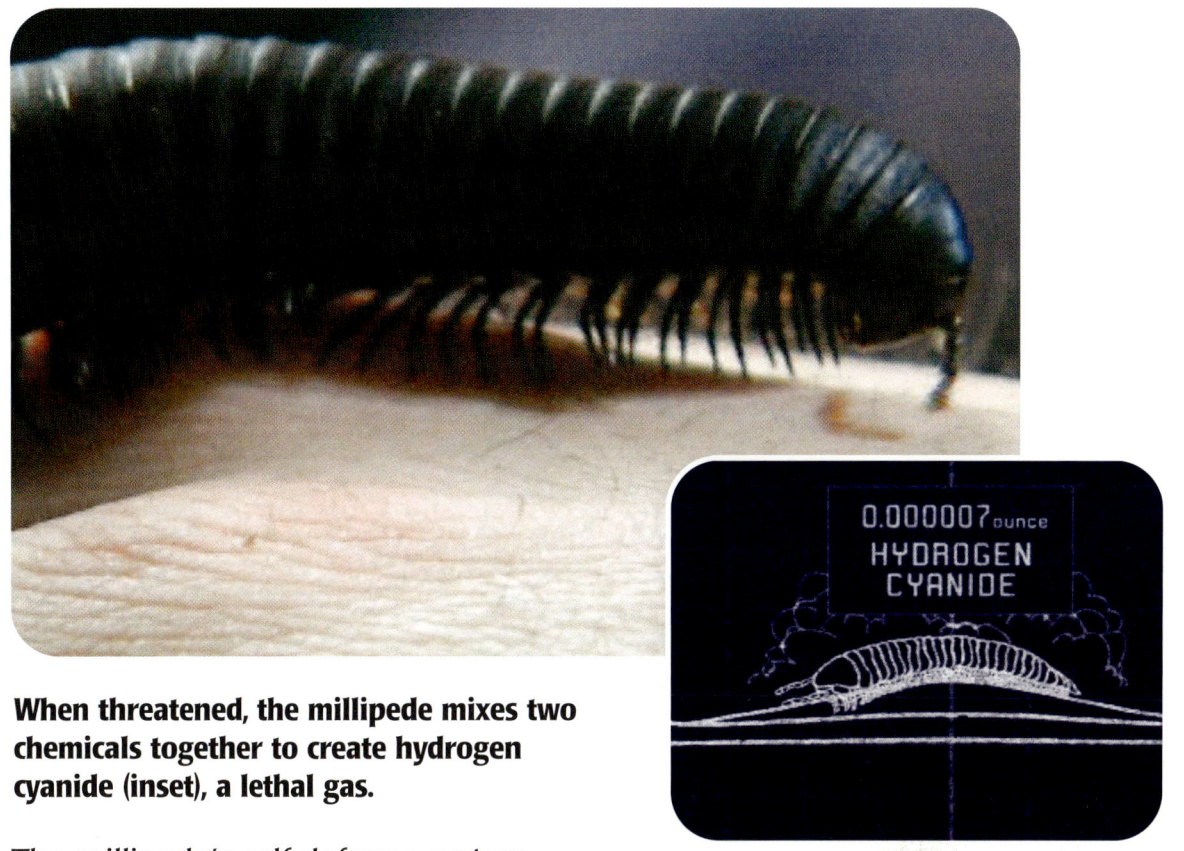

When threatened, the millipede mixes two chemicals together to create hydrogen cyanide (inset), a lethal gas.

The millipede's self-defense system would make any chemical engineer proud. When it's in danger, the millipede mixes two chemicals together in reaction chambers along the side of its body. Enzymes then convert the harmless liquid into clouds of the deadly gas hydrogen cyanide.

One millipede is capable of storing enough reactants to form seven-millionths of an ounce of hydrogen cyanide, which is enough to kill animals as large as mice. That means three hundred millipedes would create enough deadly gas to kill a human!

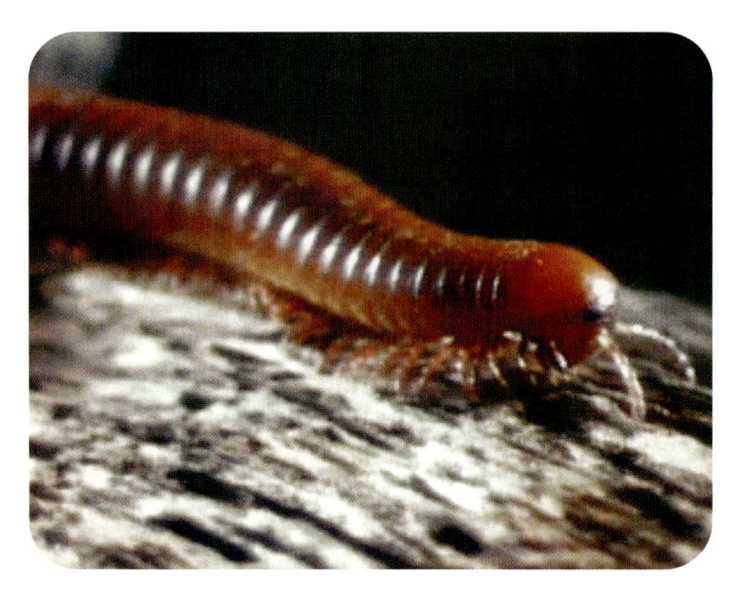

It takes a lot for a millipede to make hydrogen cyanide. A millipede would rather run than make a stink.

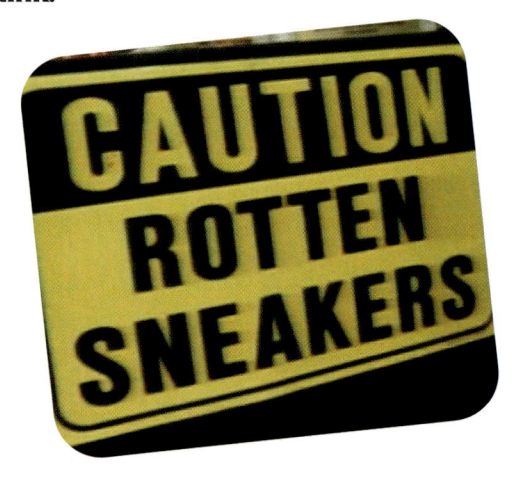

Millipedes are number three in the countdown because no other animal makes such a lethal stink. But hydrogen cyanide is exhausting to make, so a millipede would rather run than reek. It certainly has the foot power to make a speedy getaway. With hundreds of limbs, it's a good thing millipedes don't suffer from smelly feet—unlike some humans.

According to a recent survey, one in five Americans admits to sometimes having smelly feet. But not everyone has a problem with stinky feet. Every year, in Montpelier, Vermont, foul feet are celebrated in the annual International Rotten Sneaker Contest.

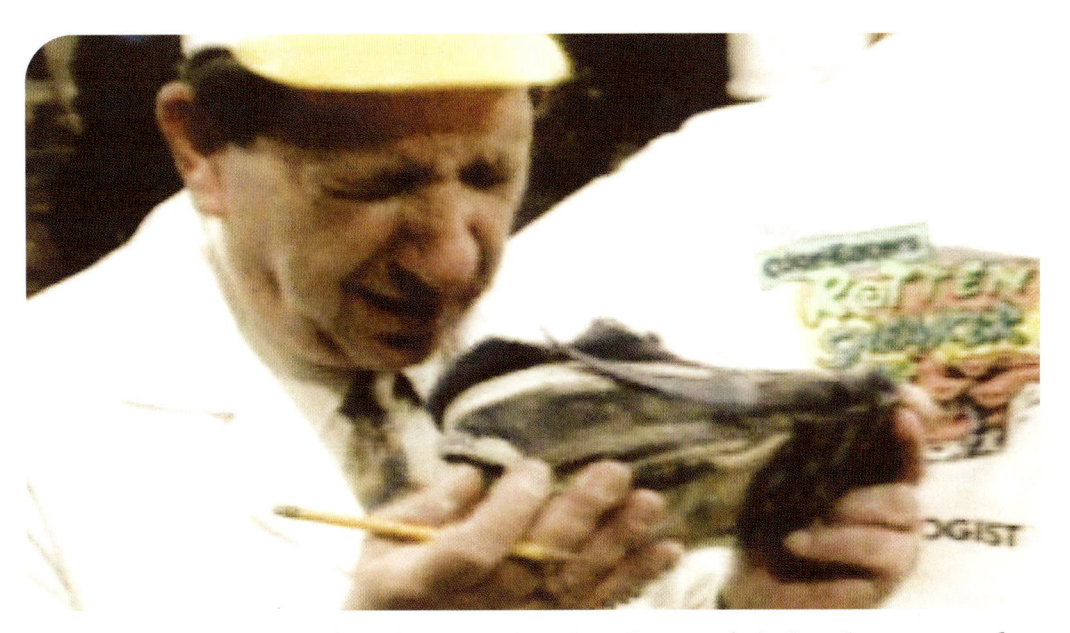

A judge at the International Rotten Sneaker Contest inhales the aroma of a sneaker past its prime.

Dozens of kids and their sweat-soaked sneakers compete for the top prize. Every year the winning sneakers are enshrined in the Hall of Fumes—a hermetically sealed trophy case where they can decompose with honor.

The millipede doesn't need to take off sneakers to make a stink, because when it comes to olfactory assaults, these guys can sock it to you naturally. But if stinky millipedes make you sick, you just won't believe what's hurled at you by our next contender.

2 The Petrel

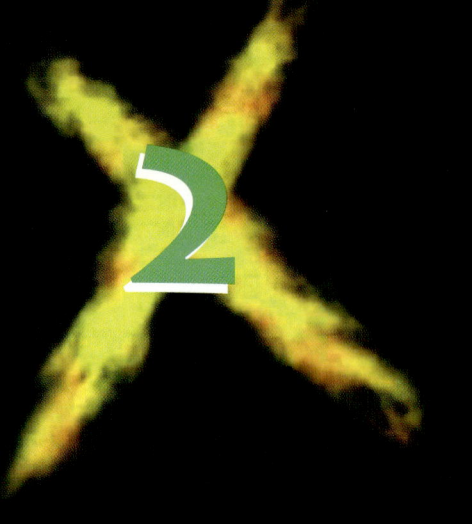

There's something very rotten in the Southern Ocean. Our next contender thinks that decay smells delicious. Diving into number two in the countdown is the giant petrel. This huge bird has such revolting personal habits that sailors call it "The Stinker"!

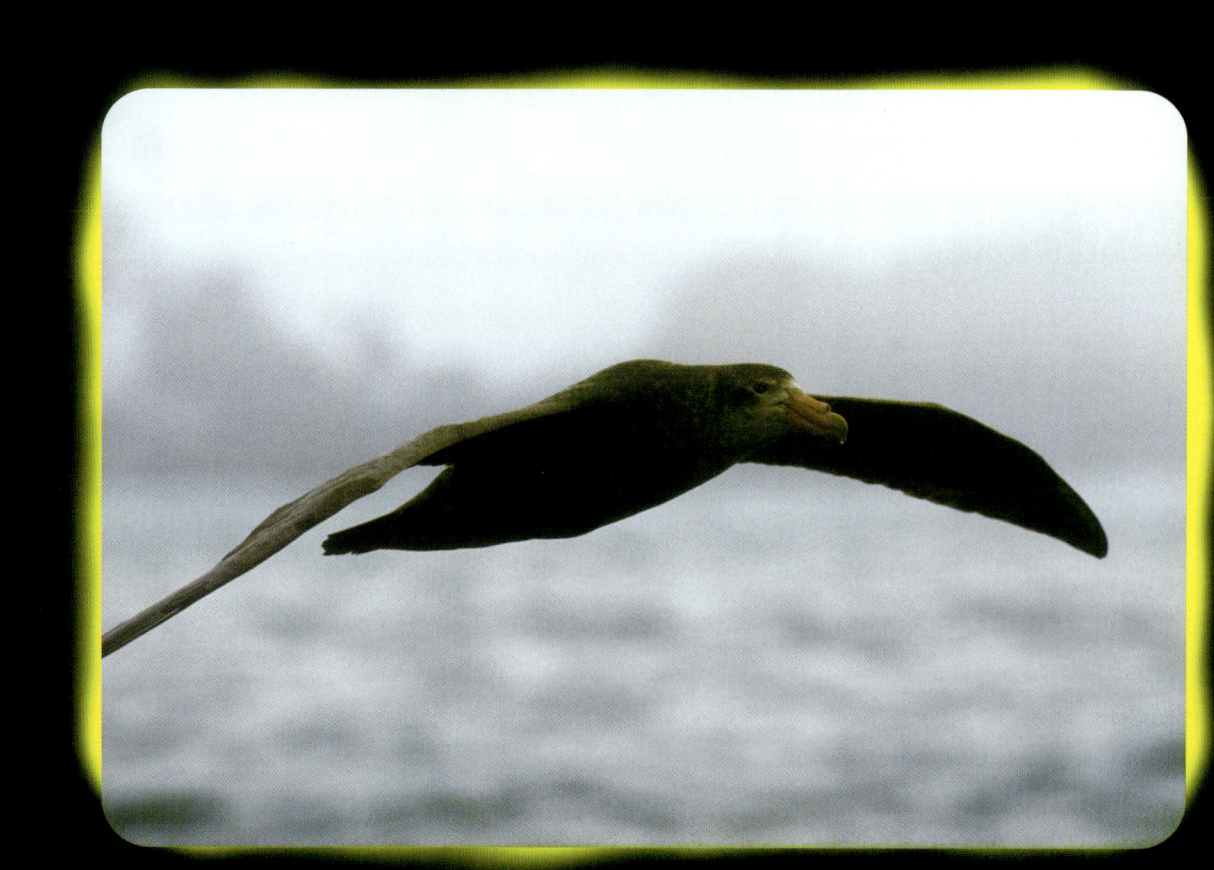

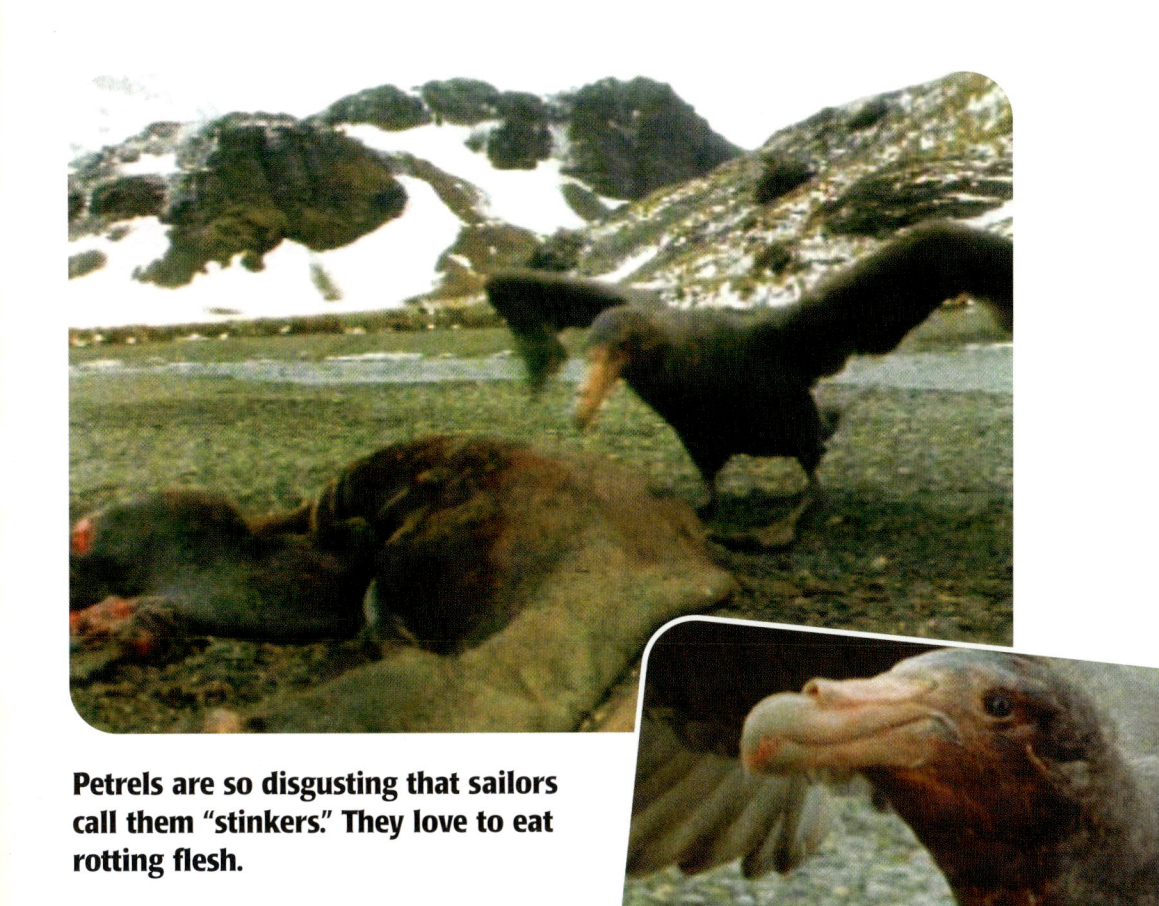

Petrels are so disgusting that sailors call them "stinkers." They love to eat rotting flesh.

Stinkers are the vultures of the southern seas. They'll eat anything rotten. But this putrid diet is only one reason why a stinker stinks. This smelly scavenger has a secret weapon.

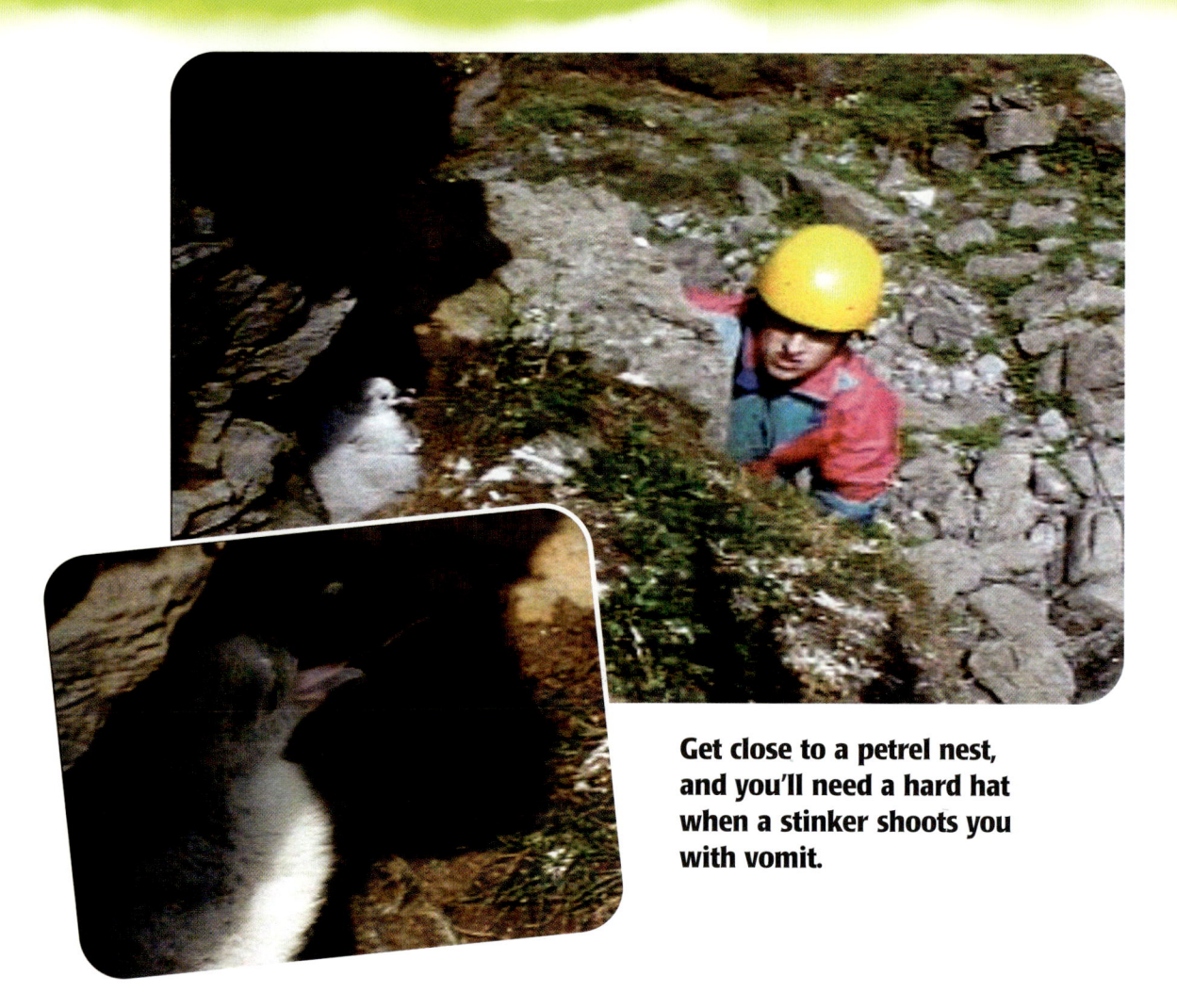

Get close to a petrel nest, and you'll need a hard hat when a stinker shoots you with vomit.

Climb too close to nesting petrels and you can get a very nasty surprise. The stinker's projectile vomit smells disgusting and is so acidic that it eats through the waterproof coating on feathers no matter how hard you try to wash it off. But stinkers aren't the only ones to use foul smells as weapons.

In World War II, the French Resistance was looking for a way to harass the invading Germans. So its American allies developed a highly secret, highly stinky weapon. It was a chemical to put into stink bombs designed to be thrown at German officers. Unfortunately, things didn't quite work out. The mixture was so unstable that it would often leave whole towns soaked in the stench.

Perhaps the French Resistance may have been better off using the projectile weapons of the stinker, or even arming itself with the animal that's number one in the countdown.

To harass invading Nazi soldiers during World War II, the French used a smelly chemical in stink bombs.

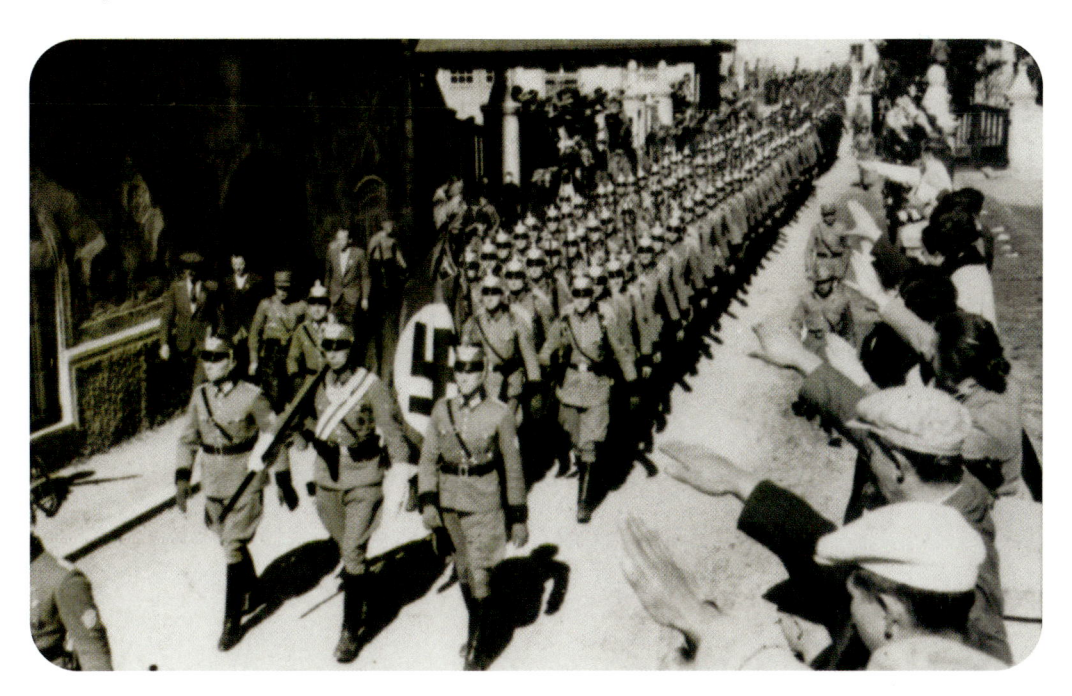

1 The Skunk

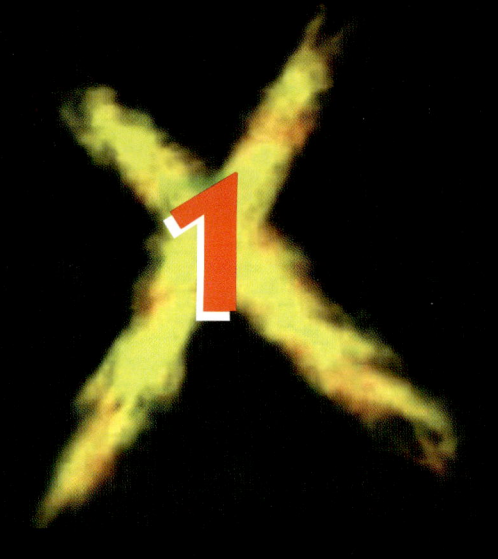

We've tracked the most extreme stinker in the countdown to this home in Orlando, Florida. Of course, it's the skunk. Jamie Kinser shares her home with not one, but eleven of the world's most extreme stinkers.

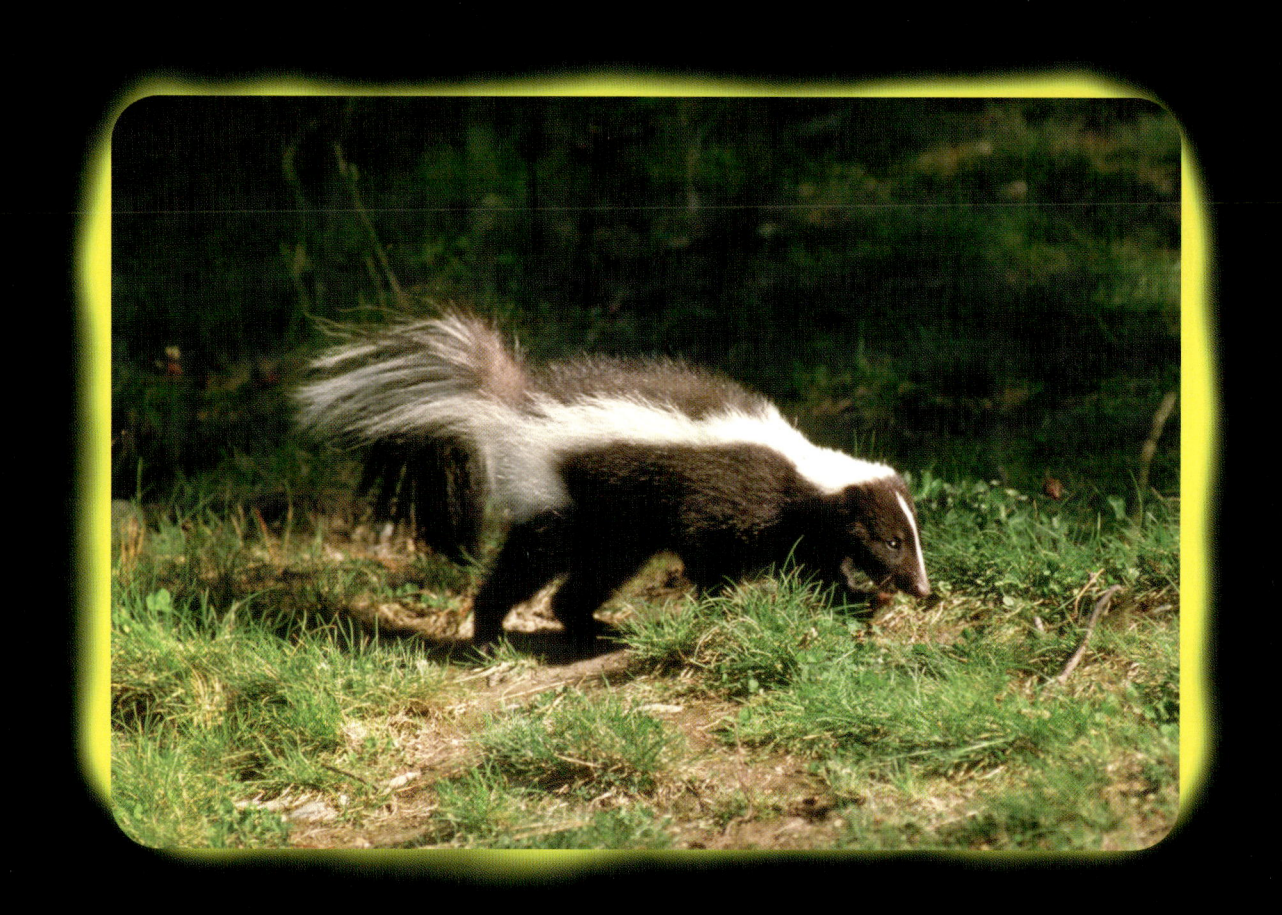

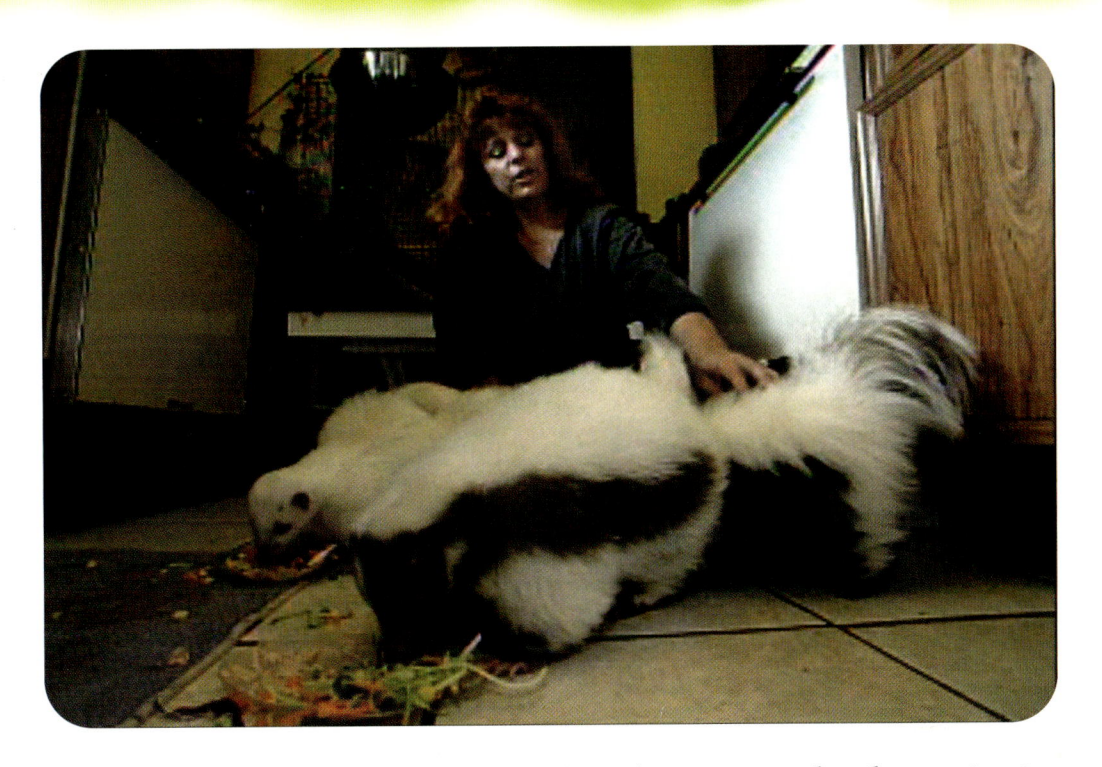

Skunks whose odor-producing glands have been removed make great pets for some people.

Why would anyone want to live with so many skunks? Kinser explains:

> They're cuddly, quiet, and clean. They're very social animals. I started out with one but it's like having potato chips—you can't just have one.

There may be up to 5 million pet skunks in America today. Professional breeders meet the demand by supplying skunks whose scent glands have been surgically removed. So while there are no stink bombs in the Kinser house, even Jamie admits that wild skunks can be real stinkers.

It's probably one of the worst smells in the world—it can bring tears to your eyes. It blinds you. It's hard to explain exactly what it does smell like. It's one of the worst things you can possibly smell other than something dead.

So what is the worst smell in the world? A nationwide survey of Americans tried to find out. Offensive bathroom odors were ranked in fourth place by 38 percent of respondents. Then came the smell of dirty diapers. Rotten eggs got 47 percent of the vote. But the clear winner, according to 60 percent of all people polled, was the skunk.

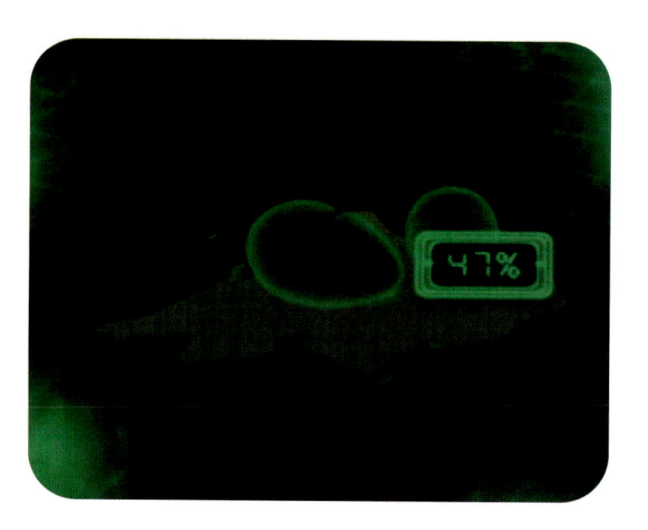

In a survey, Americans chose rotten eggs as the second worst smell in the world. The skunk's extreme odor won first place.

The skunk is number one in the countdown thanks to two walnut-sized scent glands. Even baby skunks are armed and dangerous. If you're sprayed, people over 1.5 miles downwind will be able to smell you! And the skunk's sulfurous cocktail actually sticks to you, because one chemical in the spray attaches to the proteins in hair and wool. Another ingredient reacts with the water in your sweat, so you keep stinking for days.

Why do skunks have such smelly superpowers? Most predators learn the hard way. The skunk's two scent glands are powerful guns, capable of squirting up to fifteen feet. If it misses with the first shot, it can fire again up to six times before it runs out of its stinky ammunition. No wonder scientists are taking a closer look at the skunk's smelly six-shooter.

Size is no match for the skunk's powerful squirt-gun glands, which can spray up to fifteen feet.

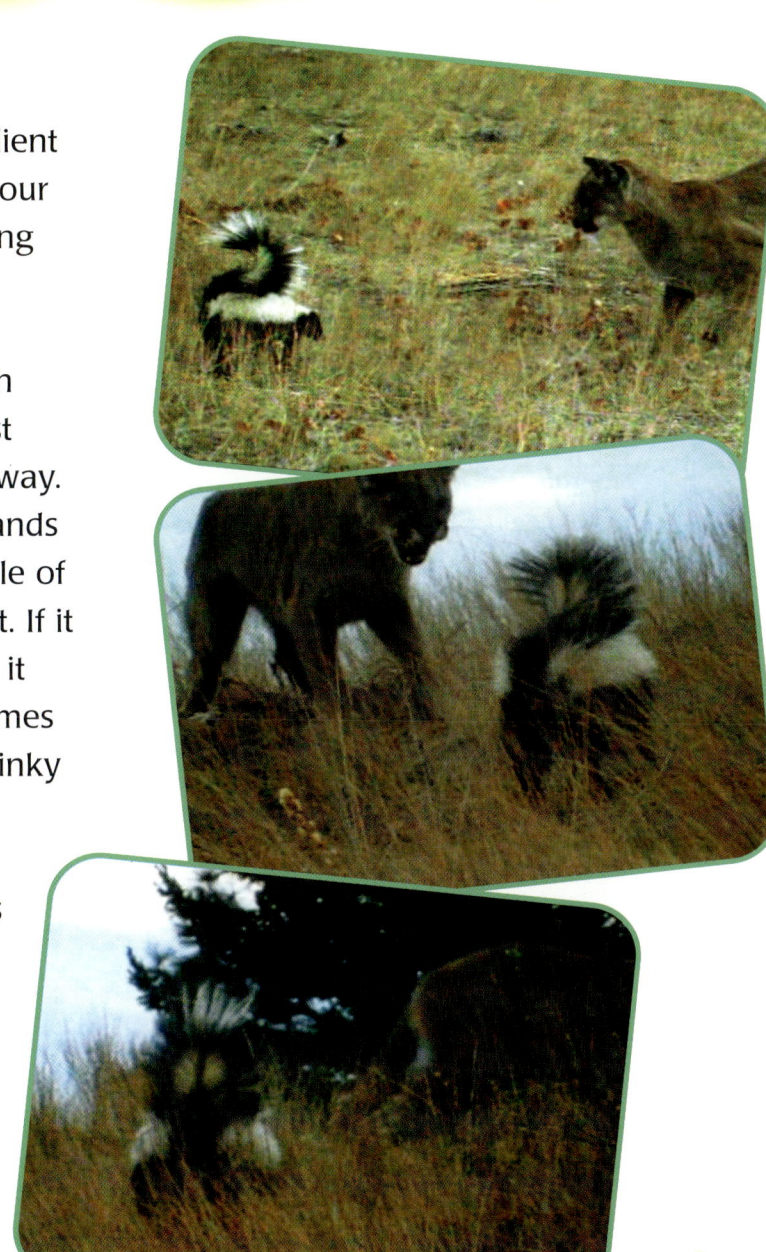

At the Monell Chemical Senses Center in Philadelphia, a team of researchers are really getting up people's noses in their search for the mother of all stink bombs. To sniff out the most universally despised odors in the world, brave volunteers are exposed to a range of disgusting smells. Their reactions are scientifically monitored from the safety of another chamber. A volunteer described how bad one smell was:

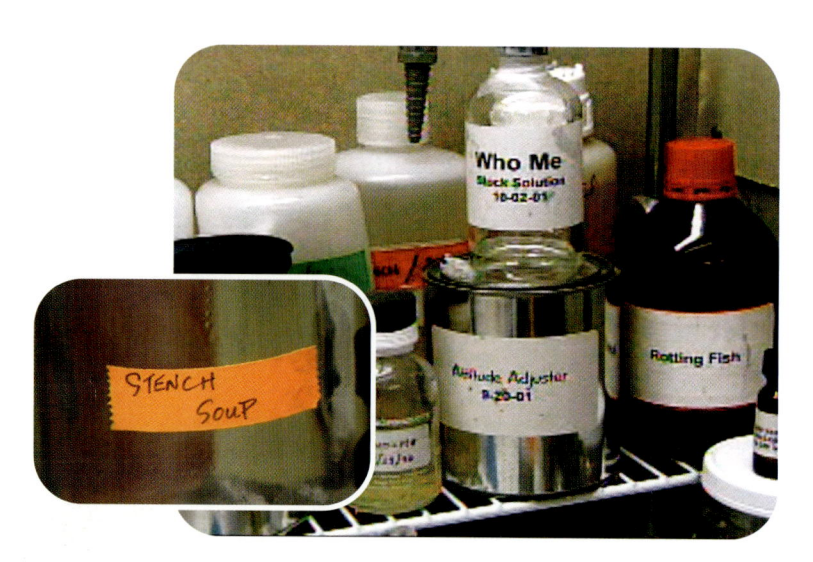

No, these aren't new perfume ideas. They are manufactured smells, the worst of which is "stench soup."

> *It was absolutely foul. As far as what it smelled like it was hard to describe—trash left out in the sun for a few days combined with a bathroom odor. It's like you took a dead cat and put it in a bag and left it in the sun for like a week.*

It's actually a concoction called "stench soup," which is the worst smell in the world, according to researcher Pam Dalton.

Stench soup was sort of an accident. We needed to dispose of many of our chemicals, and we found that when we were mixing two of our worst malodors, the human waste odor and the rotting flesh odor, the disposal bottle actually smelled a lot worse than the two of them independently. Stench seems to be a good way to describe it.

It's hoped that stench soup may one day provide the ultimate in non-lethal crowd control. Imagine dropping a stink bomb that will disperse rioters and empty streets.

A skunk already knows how to clear the street. That's why if you come across a skunk, it pays to stand clear. Because when it comes to stinks, the skunk really is The Most Extreme!

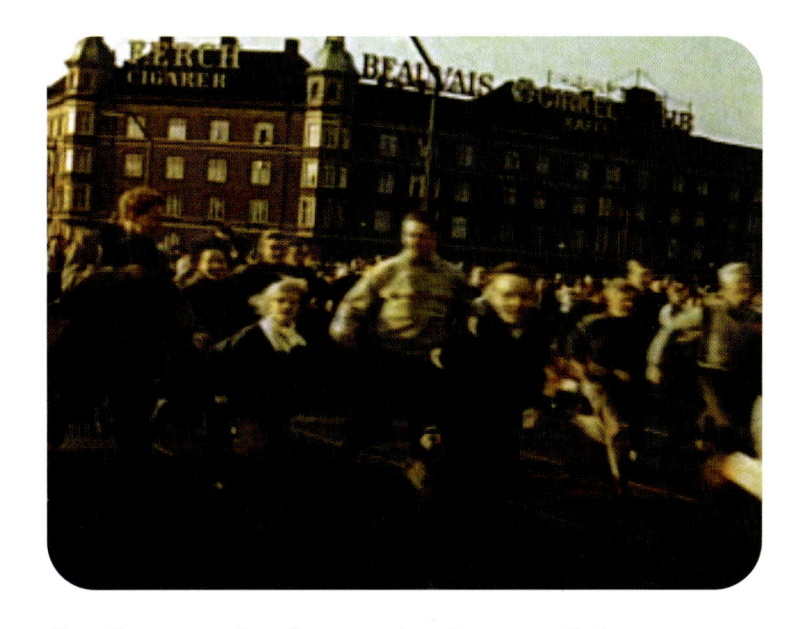

Are they running from a stench soup stink bomb? One day the foul soup may be used for crowd control.

For More Information

Melissa Cole, *Elephants*. San Diego: Blackbirch, 2003.

Theresa Greenaway, *Centipedes and Millipedes*. Chicago: Raintree, 2000.

Lee Jacobs, *Skunk*. San Diego: Blackbirch, 2002.

Jinny Johnson, *Vultures*. Chicago: Raintree, 2003.

Deborah Kops, *Vultures*. San Diego: Blackbirch, 2000.

Sally Morgan, *Hyenas*. Chicago: Raintree, 2003.

Ian Redmond, *Eyewitness: Elephant*. New York: DK, 2000.

Frank J. Staub, *Sea Lions*. Minneapolis, MN: Lerner, 2000.

Glossary

enzyme: a protein produced by living cells that helps certain biological processes

fermenting: chemically changing due to enzymes

halitosis: bad breath

molecule: the smallest particle of a substance, composed of two or more atoms

olfactory: related to the sense of smell

pheromones: chemicals produced by animals that stimulate or attract other animals

placebo: an inactive substance compared to drugs in clinical tests

savanna: treeless grassland

testosterone: a hormone that produces male secondary sex characteristics

Index

ammonia, 11
antiperspirants, 10

bacteria, 10, 11, 14, 18
bad breath, 16, 17, 18, 19
bathroom odors, 42

communication, 21
crowd control, 45

deodorant, 10
digestive gases, 14
dirty diapers, 42
dog, 4–7
"dung showering," 13

eggs, rotten, 42
elephant, 28–31

feces, 9
feet, smelly, 34
fermentation, 13
food, rotting, 18

garlic, 14
gas, 14, 18

hippopotamus, 12–15
hydrogen cyanide, 33–34
hyena, 20–23

International Rotten Sneaker Contest, 34–35

millipede, 32–35

musk ox, 24–27
musth, 29–30

nasal passages, 5
nose, 5

onions, 14

perfume, 24–25, 26, 31
petrel, 36–39
pheromones, 30, 31
projectile vomit, 38

scent glands, 41, 42–43
sea lion, 16–19
self-defense system, 33
skunk, 40–43, 45
smell, sense of, 6–7
Smell-O-Vision, 22–23
sneakers, 34–35
"stench soup," 44
stink bombs, 39, 45
sulphur, 14, 18
sweat, 9, 10

testosterone, 29–30
throwing up, 19

urine, 7, 9, 11, 25, 26

vomit, 19, 38
vulture, 8–11, 37

wolf, 5

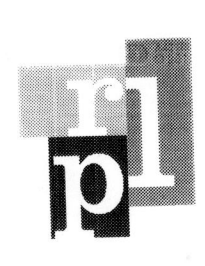

ROCKFORD PUBLIC LIBRARY